Atlas of
Osteoarthritis

A slide atlas of osteoarthritis based on the
material in this book is also available. Further
information regarding the **Slide Atlas of
Osteoarthritis** may be obtained from:

Gower Medical Publishing
101 Fifth Avenue
New York, NY 10003

Atlas of
Osteoarthritis

Allen D. Meisel, MD
Consultant in Rheumatology
Hospital for Joint Diseases –
Orthopaedic Institute
Assistant Clinical Professor of Medicine
Mount Sinai School of Medicine
New York

Peter G. Bullough, MB, ChB
Chief of Orthopedic Pathology
Hospital for Special Surgery
Professor of Pathology
Cornell University Medical College
New York

Radiologic Contributions by
Jack Twersky, MD
Associate Professor of Clinical Radiology
Downstate Medical Center
Brooklyn, NY

Foreword by
Alfred Jay Bollet, MD
Clinical Professor of Medicine
Yale University School of Medicine
Chairman, Department of Medicine
Danbury Hospital
Danbury, Connecticut

Lea & Febiger
Philadelphia

Gower Medical Publishing
New York • London

9159.

Published in North America by

Lea & Febiger
600 Washington Square
Philadelphia, PA 19106

ISBN 0-8121-0932-5 (Lea & Febiger)
ISBN 0-912143-03-7 (Gower)

Library of Congress Cataloging in Publication Data
Meisel, Allen D.
  Atlas of osteoarthritis.

  Bibliography: p.
  Includes index.
  1. Osteoarthritis – Atlases. I. Bullough, Peter G.
[DNLM: 1. Osteoarthritis – Atlases. WE 17 M515a]
RC931.067M45 1984   616.7'22   83-25344

Project Editor: Abe Krieger
Art Director: Keith Stout
Illustrators: Heather Drake
              Diane Foug

Printed in Hong Kong by Mandarin Offset International Ltd.

Preface

The **Atlas of Osteoarthritis** is designed to provide both clinician and student with a comprehensive review of osteoarthritis, linking together pathologic, radiologic, and clinical aspects of the disease to give a total picture of one of the most common afflictions of mankind. It should serve as a source book for clinical materials as it relates to current concepts of pathogenesis, should supplement the clinicians' own experience, and should amplify the information to be found in standard textbooks of rheumatology.

We believe that three observations support the need for this book in the study of osteoarthritis. First, although osteoarthritis is a very common disease which is encountered regularly by internists, general practitioners, and family practitioners, most physicians practicing today have had little or no training in the diagnosis of this rheumatic disease. Second, there is a pervasive negativism about its management and prognosis. Finally, because of a usual lack of correlation between clinical and radiologic findings, either overdiagnosis or underdiagnosis commonly occurs.

Rheumatology is a relatively recent discipline, for it was not until the turn of the century that physicians recognized the distinction between inflammatory and degenerative arthritis. In the United States, particularly at the major medical centers in New York, Boston, and Baltimore, the subspecialty of rheumatology blossomed in the early 1940s. By the mid-1950s there was a growing and enthusiastic community of rheumatologists, spurred on by Kahlar Hench's dramatic studies on the use of corticosteroids in rheumatoid arthritis.

However, it has been possible to become a physician in the United States with little or no exposure to the rheumatic diseases. As recently as 1965, one's entire training in the rheumatic diseases may have consisted of a demonstration showing a patient who was severely crippled by rheumatoid arthritis. Even today a fifth of medical schools in the United States do not have a rheumatic disease section. And even in schools where there is an adequate rheumatology staff, there is relatively little time devoted to the rheumatic diseases in the medical curriculum, with much of that time devoted to the most devastating – and rarer – inflammatory arthritides. Ironically, the average physician in practice, whether he be a rheumatologist, internist, or a general or family practitioner, is likely to devote a large percentage of his or her time in the care of these patients. Indeed, complaints related to the musculoskeletal system, and specifically osteoarthritis, may account for as many as a quarter of patient visits to the physician!

For many years rheumatologists have argued the issue of nomenclature; specifically, rejecting the term "osteoarthritis" in favor of "degenerative joint disease," or "osteoarthrosis." This didactic discussion has contributed to the relative lack of clear-cut direction in diagnostic and management approaches to the patient with osteoarthritis. We prefer the term "osteoarthritis," which emphasizes the increasingly apparent inflammatory component of the disease. The concepts of age-relatedness, wear and tear, and inevitability have been so associated with osteoarthritis that both physician and patient have come to view "arthritis" in general as a hopeless situation. As a result of this negative attitude, the patient often delays consultation and appropriate treatment.

Finally, the support services that allow for appropriate diagnosis – particularly radiologic diagnosis – are frequently limited and inadequate. Furthermore, the clinician may fail to correlate the radiologic and clinical findings. Although the incidence of radiologic osteoarthritis in some joints rises to include 80 percent of the population by age 70, clinical manifestations do not occur as frequently. This discordance may result in the overuse of the term osteoarthritis to explain any pain syndrome, leading to a major misuse of this diagnostic nomenclature.

We have attempted in this book to concisely address each of the above issues as succinctly but effectively as possible.

We were fortunate to have had the help of a number of talented people in publishing this book. Many thanks go to Dr. Gary Sterba for his research assistance, and to Mary Bentley for her careful typing of manuscript. The staff of Gower Medical Publishing in the persons of editor Abe Krieger, designer Keith Stout, and illustrators Heather Drake and Diane Foug all contributed their unique expertise and are to be congratulated for their efforts.

Allen D. Meisel, MD
Peter G. Bullough, MB, ChB

Foreword

As a student of osteoarthritis, I am delighted by the publication of this volume. By far the most prevalent form of rheumatic disorder and perhaps the most common of all diseases, osteoarthritis has long been neglected. This neglect was due not to lack of interest by physicians in common diseases but rather to a lack of knowledge about the disease. There was simply nothing worth saying about osteoarthritis except that it was common, hurt, and caused disability. However, recent advances in our understanding of cartilage physiology and the pathogenesis of osteoarthritis have resulted in the development of sound principles of prevention and therapy.

This atlas, with its succinct narrative text and plethora of superb illustrations, provides an excellent review of the current state of knowledge of osteoarthritis. Aimed at the practicing clinician as well as the medical student, it thoroughly covers the clinical, radiologic, and differential diagnostic features of the disease on a joint by joint basis. The integration of photomicrographs with clinical and radiographic views will be appreciated by the reader, for in studying osteoarthritis, it is very important to be able to visualize the lesion and then compare the pathology to the radiologic finding. The beautiful schematic illustrations clarify many important clinical points and add to the value of this volume. The introductory chapters provide a basic understanding of cartilage morphology and physiology, the biochemical and metabolic aspects of pathogenesis, mechanisms of proteoglycan degradation, and the etiologic factors that influence the extent of disease manifestation.

In recent years osteoarthritis has become even more of a concern because of the extra strain placed on the joints by the national trend toward increased physical fitness. Exercise in moderation is healthy, but the strain on individual body parts – the musculoskeletal system in particular – is often neglected due to concern for the more dramatic problems of cardiovascular and pulmonary disease. Many joggers and other exercise addicts feel that pain is "enobling" and train themselves to ignore it or "work through it." As a result, permanent joint damage is occurring with alarming frequency. Chapter 9 deals with the sports-related injuries which predispose to osteoarthritis, and in that regard is both timely and useful.

Such a volume that covers all the important features of osteoarthritis thoroughly and elegantly has long been needed. The *Atlas of Osteoarthritis* has technical and informational quality that makes it a real addition to the understanding of and to the care of patients with osteoarthritis.

Alfred Jay Bollet, MD
Clinical Professor of Medicine
Yale University School of Medicine
Chairman, Department of Medicine
Danbury Hospital

Contents

3 Osteoarthritis of the Hand

4 Osteoarthritis of the Hip

5 Osteoarthritis of the Knee

6 Osteoarthritis of the Foot

1
General Considerations in Osteoarthritis

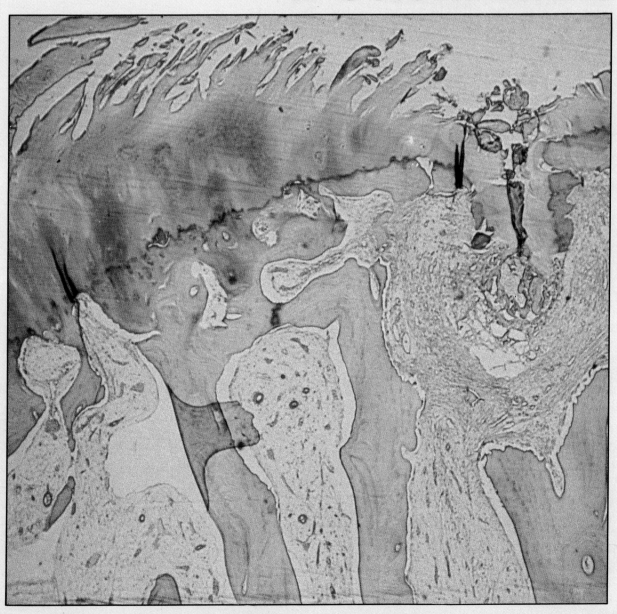

Osteoarthritis is generally regarded as a non-inflammatory disorder of movable joints characterized by functional deterioration, abrasion of articular cartilage, and formation of new bone at and around the joint surfaces. The terms degenerative joint disease, osteoarthrosis, and arthrosis are used synonymously with osteoarthritis to imply that osteoarthritis is not an inherently inflammatory process. However, since the term osteoarthritis is so well-established in the literature and since an inflammatory component has become more apparent, we will continue to use the term here.

Although there is pathologic evidence that osteoarthritis is an ancient disease (it has been identified in the bony remains of prehistoric animals as well as in early man), the term osteoarthritis was first introduced in 1890 by Sir Archibald E. Garrod. In 1909, Nichols and Richardson distinguished on the basis of anatomic features the two major categories of chronic arthritis by separating inflammatory arthritis from degenerative arthritis. "These joint lesions can be divided with great definiteness into two pathological groups. 1. Those which arise from primary proliferative changes in the joints, chiefly in the synovial membrane and in the perichondrium. 2. Those which arise primarily as a degeneration of the joint cartilage....These two pathological groups are characterized by distinct gross and histological differences." They went on to point out that "a given cause in either of the two pathological types may produce a considerable variety of different appearances, while at the same time a number of different causes may lead to the same end result in either type."

Today, osteoarthritis is the most common rheumatic disease, affecting an estimated 40.5 million adults in the United States alone. It is generally a benign disease, with less than 15 percent of those affected displaying serious symptoms or disability. Studies have shown that osteoarthritis accounts for the greatest loss of time from work in the United States and Great Britain. Thus, the disease has a considerable socioeconomic impact as well.

In this chapter, we will consider the anatomic and functional features of the normal joint; the chemistry, morphology, and physiology of the articular cartilage; the morbid anatomy and altered chemistry of the arthritic joint; and etiologic factors in the development of osteoarthritis.

THE NORMAL JOINT

The diarthrodial joint should be regarded as an organized system whose function is to provide freedom of motion, stability during motion, and an equitable distribution of load across the joint surface (Fig. 1.1). These functions in turn depend upon three structural features of the joint: first, the geometry of the articulating surfaces; second, the functional and anatomic integrity of the surrounding supportive structures (i.e., ligaments, tendons, muscles); and third, the material properties (i.e., the strength, resilience, and elasticity of the articular cartilage and the underlying subchondral bone).

The shapes of the opposing surfaces of healthy animal joints are precisely matched to allow transmission of the expected loads at the lowest and most uniform pressure. Therefore,

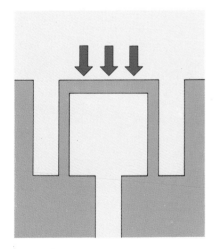
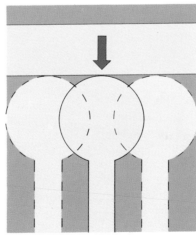
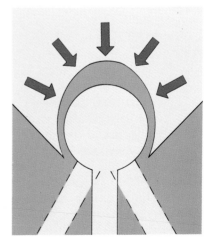

Figure 1.1   These diagrams illustrate how the shape of the joint affects function. In the configuration at left, the joint is entirely stable but unmovable. In the center diagram, the joint is freely movable but is unstable. However the most functional configuration is illustrated at right. Here, the joint is not only movable and stable but also distributes load equitably, starting at the margins of the joint and extending over the entire surface as the load increases.

any change in shape predisposes to joint surface failure. For example, meniscectomy will eventually result in the development of osteoarthritis in the compartment from which the meniscus was removed. Likewise, fractures which involve the articular surface and result in displacement often lead to osteoarthritis. In Paget's disease, the abnormal bone modeling will lead to a change in the shape of the joint and also result in osteoarthritis.

The articular surfaces of a joint can only match if they are held together in the proper relationship. A malposition of the two surfaces in relation to one another will have the same effect as an alteration in their surface shapes. Since it is the arrangement of the capsule, ligaments, tendons, etc. which mainly controls the position of the articular surfaces, damages to the soft tissue may also initiate secondary osteoarthritis. Alterations in the stiffness or resilience of the cartilage and/or bone, such as may occur, for example, in ochronosis, will also eventually result in secondary osteoarthritis.

Because of the extremely low coefficient of friction at the articular surfaces, the loads are transmitted from one surface to the other almost entirely by compression. The expanded cancellous structure of the epiphyseal end of the bone is well-suited for the transmission of compressive loads and may be contrasted with the dense cortical structure of the tubular diaphysis which has to resist bending and rotary stress as well as compression.

The expanded cancellous end of the bone is covered by a thin layer of articular cartilage which is tethered to the jagged surface of the underlying bone by a thin layer of calcified cartilage that interlocks with the bone (Fig. 1.2). Ultimately, it is the articular cartilage which bears the brunt of alterations in shape and supporting structure, and is the key to understanding osteoarthritis. As William Hunter noted in 1743, "The articulating cartilages are most happily contrived to all purposes of motion in those parts. By their uniform surface, they move upon one another with ease: by their soft, smooth and slippery surface, mutual abrasion is prevented: by their flexibility, the contiguous surfaces are constantly adapted to each other, and the friction diffused equally over the whole: by their elasticity, the violence of any shock, which may happen in running, jumping, etc., is broken and gradually spent; which must have been extremely pernicious, if the hard surfaces of bones had been immediately contiguous."

Cartilage: Chemistry, Morphology, and Physiology

Articular cartilage is composed mainly of a functional matrix having a small number of cells within it which are responsible for synthesis and maintenance. These cells represent less than 1 percent of the total volume of the cartilage.

The cellular matrix of cartilage is composed of three substances: (1) collagen, a fibrous protein that contributes to the structure and shape of cartilage; (2) proteoglycans, a glycoprotein "stuffing material" found between collagen fibrils that confers stiffness and elasticity to the cartilage; and (3) water (up to 80 percent of the weight of the cartilage), which contributes to the turgor of the tissue. It is this combination that gives cartilage its special properties.

Figure 1.2   Photomicrograph reveals that the cancellous end of bone is covered by a layer of articular cartilage which is fastened to the underlying bone by a thin layer of calcified cartilage. It is the articular cartilage which will be most affected by osteoarthritis.

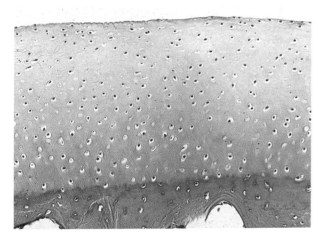

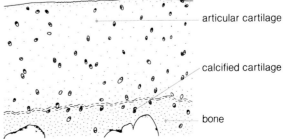

articular cartilage

calcified cartilage

bone

Collagen

Hyaline cartilage has a unique type of collagen, type II, which is structurally characterized by three alpha-1 (II) chains in its triple-helix molecule (Fig. 1.3). These chains have more hydroxyglycine residues than does type I collagen, and many of those residues are glycosylated. These biochemical characteristics are responsible for the finer diameter of collagen fibers in cartilage, which, in turn, probably affects the mechanical properties of this tissue.

In the surface layer of cartilage, the collagen fibers are closely packed, of fine diameter, and mostly oriented parallel to the joint surface (Fig. 1.4). This arrangement protects the cartilage against abrasive forces, and transmits the vertical compressive load on the surface to the joint margins in much the same way that

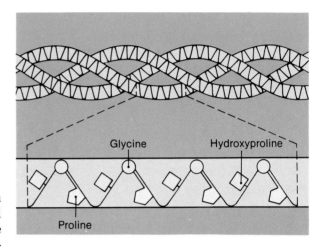

Figure 1.3 Schematic diagram shows the helical structure of type II collagen. The molecule is composed of three polypeptide chains that intertwine as a triple helix. In each chain, there is a glycine residue at every third amino acid position. Hydroxyproline frequently precedes the glycine, and proline frequently follows.

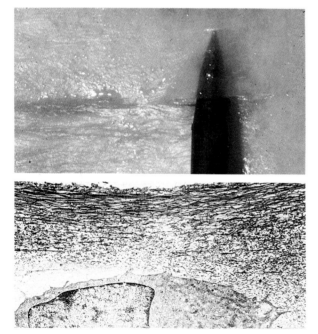

Figure 1.4 In the photograph at top, a pin can be seen elevating the surface layer of collagen. In the transmission electron micrograph at bottom, the closely packed surface layer of collagen can be appreciated, with a chondrocyte noted in the lower part of the picture.

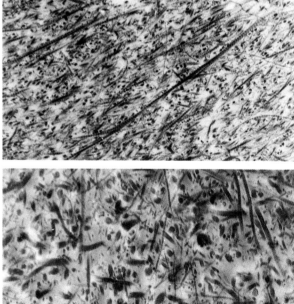

Figure 1.5 In the transmission electron micrograph at top, the surface collagen fibers are thin and closely packed electron-dense structures. In contrast, an EM taken at the same magnification but at a deeper layer (bottom) shows that the fibers are much thicker and more widely separated.

the fabric of a chair transmits vertical load onto the frame of the chair, which actually serves as the supporting structure.

The collagen content of cartilage progressively diminishes from the superficial to the deep layer (Fig. 1.5). In the deeper layers, collagen fibers are more widely separated, are thicker in diameter, and are aligned in such a fashion as to form a web of arch-shaped structures (Fig. 1.6). The fibers are continuous with those in the calcified layer of cartilage but not with the underlying subchondral bone (Fig. 1.7). The arrangement of the arches allows the collagen to constrain the proteoglycan gel which is entrapped in the matrix. The web of arches functions as a unit, and damage to one section affects the architectural integrity of the whole unit.

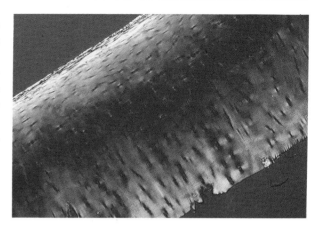

Figure 1.6   In this polarized photomicrograph, the surface collagen fibers can be visualized as blue, the deeper collagen fibers (which are perpendicular) as yellow. Collagen cannot be seen in the intermediate area because the fibers are parallel or perpendicular to the plane of polarization.

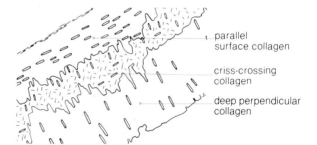

parallel
surface collagen

criss-crossing
collagen

deep perpendicular
collagen

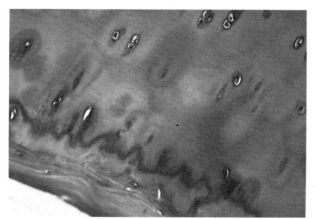

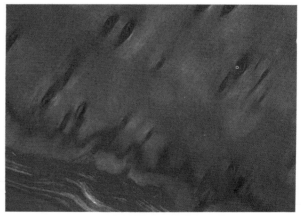

Figure 1.7   In the photomicrograph at left, one may note an irregular, serrated, basophilic line (tidemark) which demarcates the articular cartilage from the thin layer of calcified cartilage beneath. In this view, it is difficult to appreciate the junction between the calcified cartilage and the underlying bone. However, under polarized light (*right*) the subchondral bone (red) can be clearly demarcated from the overlying cartilage (blue), thus demonstrating that the cartilage and bone are discontinuous structures.

Proteoglycans

Although collagen is the major determinant of the shape and form of articular cartilage, the collagen meshwork requires the presence of proteoglycans to maintain cartilage function. These large, hydrated proteoglycan molecules surround on all sides and are loosely attached to the collagen fibrils (Fig. 1.8). In laboratory studies, when proteoglycans are enzymatically degraded with trypsin or hyaluronidase, cartilage retains its normal shape but loses its elastic properties (Fig. 1.9).

In contrast to the solid structure of collagen, proteoglycan is a sticky, gel-like molecule, with a shape analogous to a test-tube brush. These molecules are extremely hydrophilic, which accounts for the high water content in articular cartilage and, in turn, produces a high swelling pressure which provides the cartilage with its elastic resistance to compression (Fig. 1.10).

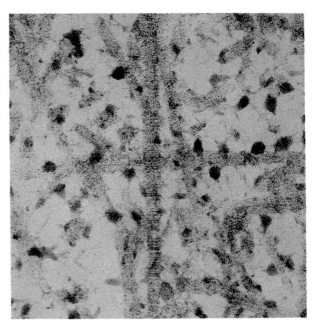

Figure 1.8 Transmission electron micrograph shows that adjacent to the surface of the collagen fibers are dye-stained black globules, representing proteoglycans.

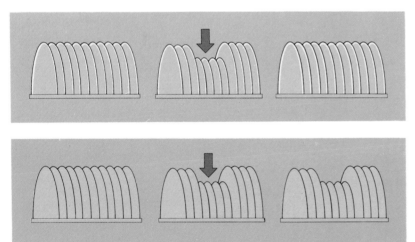

Figure 1.9 These schematic diagrams illustrate the interdependent nature of collagen and proteoglycan. Normal cartilage is represented by palisading arcades of collagen with closely associated proteoglycans. If this cartilage is deformed under pressure, it returns to its original state as soon as pressure is released due to the resiliency conferred by the proteoglycans. However, if the proteoglycans were enzymatically digested without affecting the collagen, the cartilage would, under pressure, retain its shape but lose its resiliency.

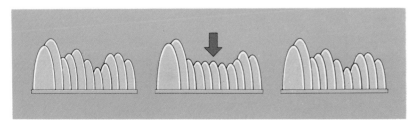

Figure 1.10 As seen in this schematic diagram, if collagen is partially digested by collagenase, the shape and the structure of the cartilage are markedly altered. However, due to the presence of proteoglycans, the cartilage retains its resiliency.

Most proteoglycan exists as enormous aggregate molecules (molecular weight of 100 million or more) consisting of a core of hyaluronic acid, link glycoproteins, and protein side chains lined with a variety of sulfated mucopolysaccharides (Fig. 1.11). These mucopolysaccharides are mainly chondroitin 4, chondroitin 6, and keratan sulfate, the relative amounts varying with the age and location of the cartilage. The proportion of chondroitin 4 sulfate is higher in children, while the proportion of keratan sulfate is higher in older individuals and in the deeper layers of the articular cartilage. The topographic distribution of proteoglycans exhibits a great deal of individual variation which may reflect local physical stresses (Fig. 1.12).

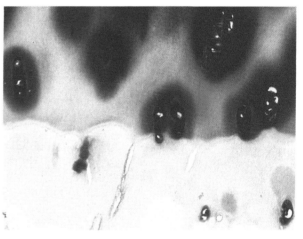

Figure 1.12   In this photomicrograph, the proteoglycans can be seen concentrating about the cells with a nonuniform distribution within the cartilage.

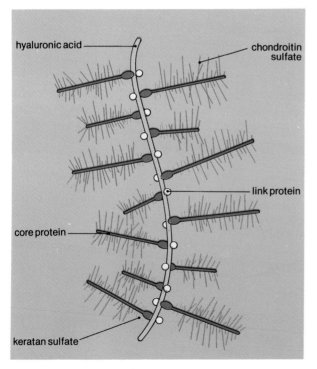

Figure 1.11   In this diagram of a proteoglycan molecule one can note a central core of hyaluronic acid and multiple side chains. Each side chain has a protein core with numerous attached mucopolysaccharides consisting principally of chondroitin sulfate and keratan sulfate.

Chondrocytes

The chondrocyte is the metabolically active cellular component of cartilage that is involved in cartilage matrix synthesis and, to some extent, breakdown (Fig. 1.13). Chondrocytes vary in size, shape, and number of cells per unit volume of tissue from the surface to the deeper layers and in different anatomic locations. It has been suggested that the latter is inversely proportional to cartilage thickness. Generally, the cells at the cartilage surface are flatter, smaller, and more closely packed than the cells deeper in the matrix. Mitochondria are sparse in cartilage cells, which probably relates to their comparatively low rates of oxygen consumption. The cells in the deeper uncalcified zone have the most prominent endoplasmic reticulum and Golgi apparatus, the cytoplasmic structures known to be associated with protein synthesis and with the sulfation of the mucopolysaccharides which line the proteoglycan side chains. Cell division

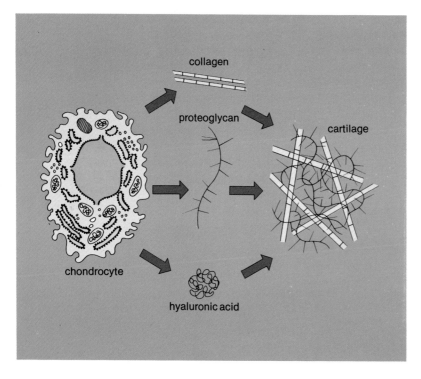

Figure 1.13 Diagrammatic representation of a chondrocyte showing its metabolic functions.

is not normally observed in adults, but does occur in response to injury or disease.

The cell membrane shows numerous short as well as some longer, branched cytoplasmic processes, but they make no connection with the processes of other chondrocytes (unlike the osteocytic processes in bone). In the extracellular matrix adjacent to the cells of adult articular cartilage and in the hypertrophic zone of the growth plate, small membrane-bound vesicles are visible (Fig. 1.14). These vesicles are believed to play an important role in the calcification of cartilage matrix.

Lipid is present in the extracellular matrix around the cells; at the surface of the articular cartilage there is a diffuse layer of extracellular lipid which may have a role in cartilage lubrication (Fig. 1.15). It has been noted that when the surface of the cartilage is wiped with a lipid solvent, the coefficient of friction of the cartilage is significantly increased.

Chondrocytes receive their nutrients from the synovial fluid. Apparently, intermittent joint motion is necessary to distribute nutrients throughout the cartilage and to remove waste materials.

Although the synthesis of collagen by chondrocytes in an immature animal can be demonstrated by the use of tritiated proline isotope, the turnover of collagen in normal adults is so slow that it cannot be measured. However, in young rabbit knee cartilage, the half-life of collagen is only a few months.

The morphology of the chondrocyte as well as its metabolic activity with regard to proteoglycan synthesis appears to be dependent upon the layer at which it is found. In the superficial layer, the cells are flat and proteoglycan synthesis is minimal. In the deep layer, the cells tend to form radial groups that follow the pattern of collagen deposition. The most intense staining for proteoglycans occurs around the chondrocyte, especially in the deep layer of cartilage (see Fig. 1.12). In the calcified layer, the cells are apparently nonviable, and the matrix is heavily calcified.

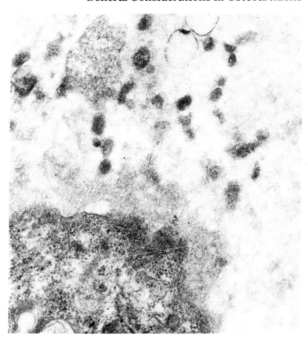

Figure 1.14 Electron micrograph demonstrates vesicles in the extracellular matrix around the chondrocyte as electron-dense particles.

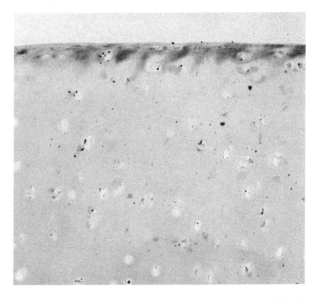

Figure 1.15 In this photomicrograph, stained with oil red O, the red staining on the surface of the cartilage represents lipid.

Enzymatic Mechanisms for the Degradation of Cartilage

Mechanisms for the degradation of collagen and proteoglycan clearly exist. Collagenase activity in normal articular cartilage has recently been demonstrated, but its role in collagen turnover remains unclear.

On the other hand, it is known that proteoglycan can be degraded by a variety of mechanisms, its molecular structure rendering it especially susceptible to degradation by proteolytic enzymes. Some of these enzymes—specifically, lysozyme, neutral proteinases,

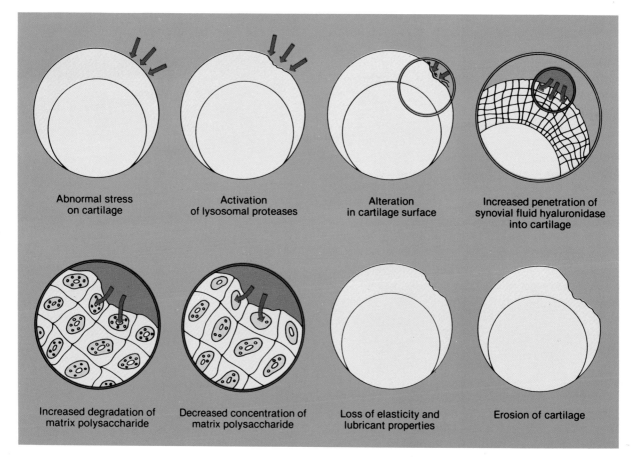

Figure 1.16   This diagram illustrates the sequence of factors leading to cartilage breakdown. (Modified from Bollet, 1967)

cathepsins (D, B1, and F) and other acid hydro-
lases – have been implicated as pathogenic factors in osteoarthritis. The degradative effects
of the neutral proteinases and cathepsins may
be balanced in vivo and modulated by small
proteins which are native to cartilage and exhibit antiproteinase activity. Hyaluronidase,
which can degrade chondroitin sulfate chains
to oligosaccharides, is present in the synovial
membrane and in synovial fluid, but has not
been found in articular cartilage.

Ultimately, the depletion of proteoglycans is
a cardinal feature of all forms of both naturally
occurring and experimental osteoarthritis.
This depletion can be demonstrated by reduced levels of hexosamine, hexuronate, and
keratan sulfate in the matrix. Under normal
conditions, the combination of proteoglycan
molecules and collagen fibers allows cartilage
to act as a molecular sieve, admitting small
molecules but excluding larger ones, especially degradative enzymes. The surface layer of
cartilage in particular, with its tightly packed
fine collagen fibers, is important in this regard.
Without its molecular sieve action, cartilage
becomes vulnerable to degradative enzymes.
The potential for cartilage destruction thus increases once a surface ulceration appears and
permits synovial fluid with its repository of
hyaluronidases and other enzymes to perme-
ate the interstitial matrix (Fig. 1.16).

THE MORBID ANATOMY OF OSTEOARTHRITIS

Whatever the cause of injury, there are certain
basic cellular and tissue responses. Histologically, there will be signs of degeneration and
signs of regeneration and/or repair.

Cartilage Injury and Repair

The earliest observable morphologic change in
osteoarthritis is the breaking up of the collagen meshwork, particularly at the surface of
the joint, giving the cartilage a rough and
shaggy appearance. This degenerative process is known as fibrillation (Fig. 1.17).

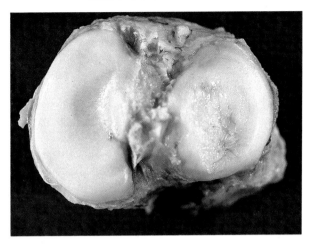

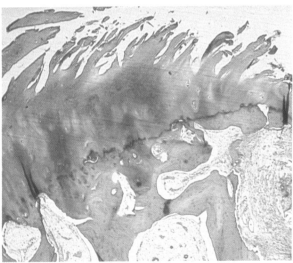

Figure 1.17 Gross pathologic photograph of a tibial plateau (*top*) clearly demonstrates the rough shaggy appearance of fibrillated cartilage of the lateral compartment. On
photomicrographic view (*bottom*), the fibrillated cartilage
surface is also evident.

Proteoglycan may also be altered, either in amount produced or by enzymatic disaggregation, resulting in cartilage softening, or chondromalacia (Fig. 1.18), and alterations in the staining properties (Fig. 1.19).

The earliest pathologic finding in progressive osteoarthritis is a disruption of the thin surface overlying the load-bearing cartilage, with flaking and pitting of the cartilage. Erosion and ulceration in some of these sites continues until the area becomes almost com-

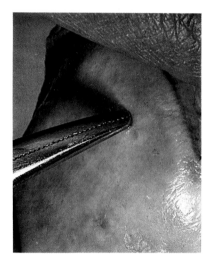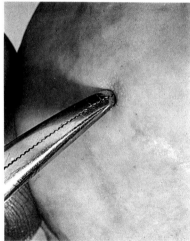

Figure 1.18   As demonstrated on the left, normal cartilage is firm but resilient and can be compressed with some degree of pressure (exerted here by a hemostat). However, as the cartilage softens or becomes chondromalacic, it also becomes palpably softer (*right*).

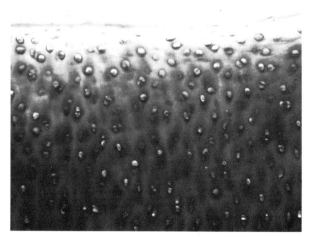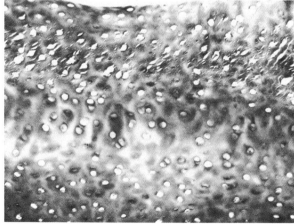

Figure 1.19   Intense staining of proteoglycan can be noted in the perichondrial area in this photomicrograph of normal cartilage (*left*). However, as the degenerative process progresses, proteoglycan loss in the matrix can be noted by the decreased intensity of the staining (*right*).

pletely denuded of cartilage. Vertical fissures may penetrate to the depth of the cartilage, and proliferative clones of the chondrocytes usually cluster around the margins of these fissures (Fig. 1.20).

Cellular injury is evident as focal cell necrosis (Fig. 1.21); occasionally, cell necrosis may be quite extensive and, rarely, all the cells are necrotic. When the latter occurs, the condition is referred to as chondrolysis and usually leads to a rapid disappearance of cartilage from the articular surfaces of a joint (Fig. 1.22).

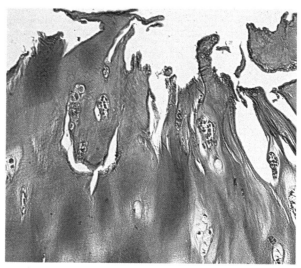

Figure 1.20   Photomicrograph demonstrates vertical fissures extending to the deep layers of the cartilage, with clones of chondrocytes at the fissure margins.

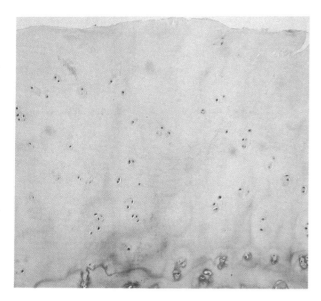

Figure 1.21   Photomicrograph demonstrates areas of cartilage with no chondrocytes, a consequence of focal cell necrosis.

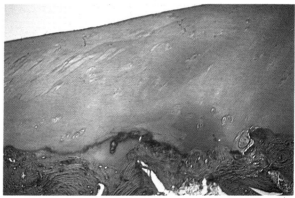

Figure 1.22   In this photomicrograph, there are no viable chondrocytes visible within the cartilage (chondrolysis), indicative of total cell death.

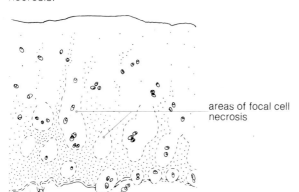

areas of focal cell necrosis

Evidence of cartilage regeneration or repair is also seen in both the cells and the matrix. In cells, this is seen as cellular proliferation forming clumps (or clones) of chondrocytes; in the matrix, this is noted by the appearance of disordered reparative collagen (Fig. 1.23).

Reparative cartilage in a damaged joint may come from either of two sites: If it comes from the damaged cartilage itself, this is regarded as intrinsic repair (Fig. 1.24), and if it comes from tissues outside the cartilage (i.e., the synovial membrane or subchondral bone), this is regarded as extrinsic repair (Fig. 1.25). In most cases of osteoarthritis, both intrinsic and extrinsic reparative cartilage may be found.

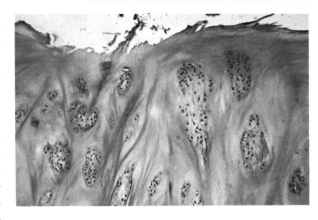

Figure 1.23 Photomicrograph of regenerating cartilage. As part of the reparative process, chondrocytes proliferate and form clumps. The collagen fibers in the matrix are also clumped and in disarray.

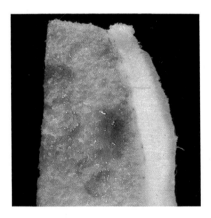 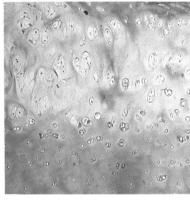 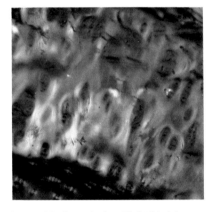

Figure 1.24 Gross specimen (*left*) demonstrates intrinsic cartilage repair, as evidenced by a white, wedge-shaped opaque area between the normal surface and the normal deeper cartilage. Photomicrograph of this area (*center*) shows proliferating cells, cellular clumping, and disarrayed collagen. Under polarized light (*right*), one can more easily see the disarrayed collagen in the central area of the cartilage.

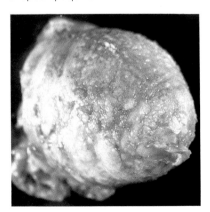 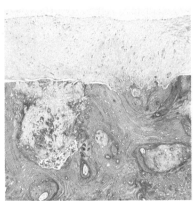

Figure 1.25 In this gross specimen of a deformed femoral head (*left*), the weight-bearing surface has been recovered with an irregular, cobblestoned layer of cartilage. A photomicrograph of this cartilage (*right*) reveals that it arises from the subchondral bone.

Bone Injury and Repair

It is important to realize that when a joint begins to break down, all the tissues are involved in the process. Osteoarthritis is, therefore, not only a disease of articular cartilage but also a disease which affects the bone, the synovial membrane, and the supportive structures around the joints.

As the articular cartilage is denuded from the articular surface, the underlying bone becomes polished or eburnated (Fig. 1.26) and is subjected to increasingly greater local stresses. As a result of this, the bone undergoes focal pressure necrosis of its superficial layer (Fig. 1.27), with consequent focal microfractures in the subchondral bone area. Sometimes, articular fractures and denudation of the cartilage lead to high intra-articular pressure which results in focal bone resorption associated with subchondral cyst formation (Fig. 1.28).

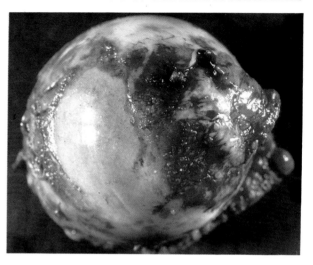

Figure 1.26   Gross superior view of a femoral head shows an area of complete cartilage loss, with polishing or eburnation of the underlying bone.

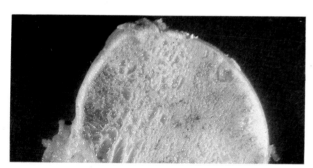

Figure 1.27   In this gross frontal section of a hip, one may note a localized area of pressure necrosis on the weight-bearing surface.

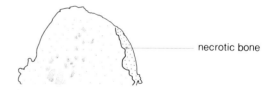

necrotic bone

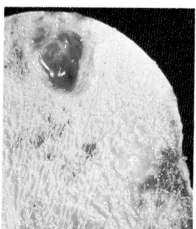

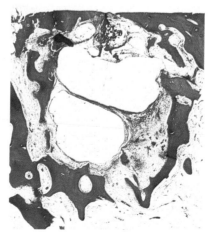

Figure 1.28   In this gross frontal section of a femoral head (left), one can see a distinct cystic lesion. Photomicrograph of tissue from the femoral head (right) shows the cyst at the surface, but entirely within the subchondral bone.

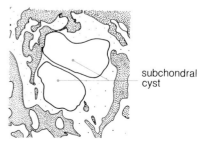

subchondral cyst

In general, subchondral cysts are only seen in the absence of overlying cartilage and represent the diffusion of synovial pressure into the subchondral bone (Fig. 1.29).

These bone injuries are followed by reparative changes: the formation of new bone on both the surface of the existing trabeculae and in the marrow spaces, resulting in bony sclerosis (Fig. 1.30).

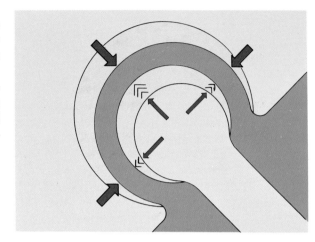

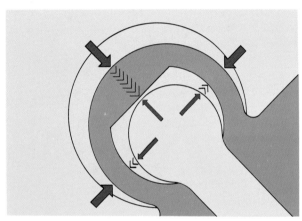

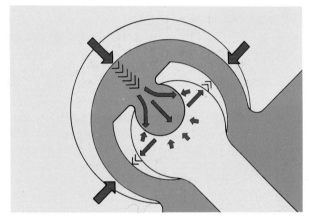

Figure 1.29   Subchondral bone cysts occur secondary to small openings at the articular surface which communicate with the joint space. In this sequence of diagrams, the large arrows represent the high synovial pressure which is normally very much greater than the infraosseous pressure (small arrows). It is this pressure gradient that is responsible for the formation of subchondral cysts. Under normal conditions (*top right*), cartilage dissipates the pressure difference between the joint space and the infraosseous bone. However, with the loss of cartilage (*left*), the intrasynovial pressure is transmitted directly to the underlying bone. Consequently, cysts form and increase in size until the pressure gradient is dissipated (*bottom right*).

Figure 1.30   Photomicrograph shows extensive subchondral sclerosis and new bone formation at the joint surface (eburnation).

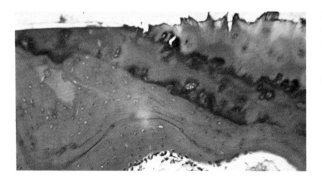

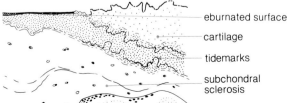

eburnated surface

cartilage

tidemarks

subchondral sclerosis

Synovial Membrane Injury

Breakdown of cartilage and bone will result in an increased amount of debris in the joint cavity; this debris is removed by the phagocytic cells (A cells) of the synovial membrane. As a result, the synovial membrane becomes both hypertrophic and hyperplastic (Fig. 1.31). It has been shown in experimental animals that the injection of hyaluronic acid into the joint cavity produces an inflammatory change in the synovial membrane. For this reason, some degree of chronic inflammation may be expected, especially with rapid breakdown of the articular components.

Histologic studies have shown an overlap between osteoarthritis and rheumatoid arthritis with regard to the histologic parameters of inflammation (Fig. 1.32). Furthermore, in osteoarthritis, extension of the hyperplastic synovium onto the articular surface of the joint (particularly in the hip) is a common find-

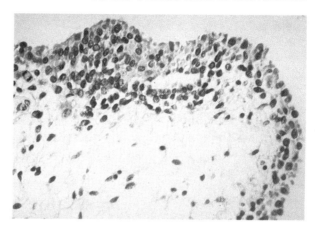

Figure 1.31 Photomicrograph of the synovial membrane from a patient with osteoarthritis shows a markedly hyperplastic synovium with mild chronic inflammatory cell infiltrate.

Figure 1.32 The extent of pannus in the hip of patients with osteoarthritis ( ) as compared to rheumatoid arthritis ( ). Note the degree of overlap with regard to the number of patients showing 10 percent coverage of the femoral head with pannus.

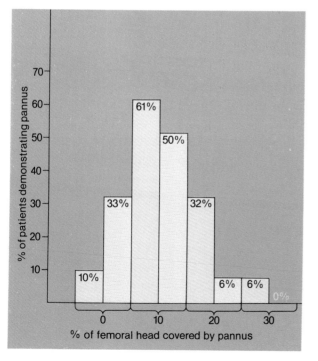

ing (Fig. 1.33). However, the extent of this pannus and its aggressiveness are much less extensive than that seen in patients with rheumatoid arthritis.

The hypertrophied and hyperplastic synovium is also likely to be damaged as the increased amount of synovial tissue extends into the joint cavity and is traumatized. Evidence of bleeding into the joint with subsequent hemosiderin staining of the synovial membrane is a common finding and may occasionally be marked. When this is the case, the orange-brown staining of the synovium seen at operation should not be confused with pigmented villonodular synovitis.

Since, under normal circumstances, the synovial membrane is responsible for the nutrition of the articular cartilage, it may be expected that the chronically inflamed and scarred synovial membrane of chronic osteoarthritis may not function in this regard, thereby contributing to the chronicity of the arthritic process.

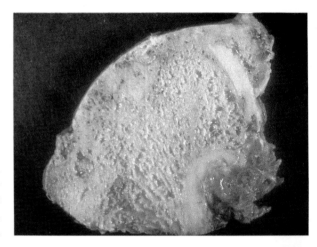

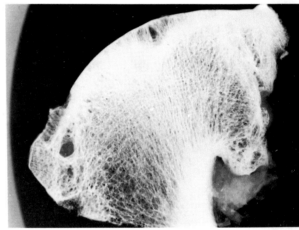

Figure 1.34   Gross frontal section of the femoral head (*top*) reveals large osteophytes at the medial and lateral surfaces, both actually becoming a part of the weight-bearing articulation. Radiograph (*bottom*) demonstrates the extent of subchondral sclerosis and subchondral cyst formation. (The dotted line in the accompanying diagram represents the original shape of the joint.)

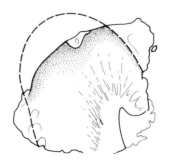

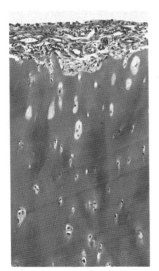
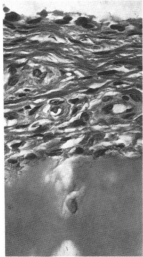

Figure 1.33   Low-power photomicrograph of cartilage (*left*) shows a hyperplastic, fibrous synovial membrane overlying the surface of the cartilage (pannus). On high-power view (*right*) it can be noted that the synovium is fibrovascular, with relatively few inflammatory cells.

Injury and Repair of the Joint as a Whole

While the degenerative process is important, it should also be noted that morphologic repair of the joint occurs at the same time. In the reparative process there is restoration of joint shape, the redistribution of load over the surfaces, and restoration of stability. The most obvious way in which this restoration is achieved is through the production of new bone in various locations along the joint surface, and particularly at the margins of the joint.

Remodeling of bone occurs concomitant with early osteoarthritis, resulting in subchondral bone thickening and formation of marginal new bone in the shape of spurs. These pieces of reparative bone are referred to as osteophytes (Fig. 1.34). In the advanced stages of osteoarthritis, the remodeling is considerable, as is the gross overall deformity including subluxation, instability, and the appearance of "joint mice" (loose bodies within the articular space). In advanced lesions, there is bone-on-bone contact, with eburnated subchondral bone exposed to the joint space (Fig. 1.35).

It should be pointed out that the relationship between these secondary reparative changes and the degenerative changes of osteoarthritis is still not entirely clear. Indeed, osteophytes have been found to develop even when the cartilage remains essentially normal. Clinical evidence to date suggests that the presence of osteophytes in the knee and hip does not always herald the development of symptomatic osteoarthritis, and radiographic studies have shown that two-thirds of knees with evidence of osteophyte formation do not develop the degenerative changes of osteoarthritis, even when followed for as long as 17 years. The chronicity of osteoarthritis is probably the result of the chronicity of the injuries and should not be regarded as a failure on the part of the tissues at the joint to repair themselves.

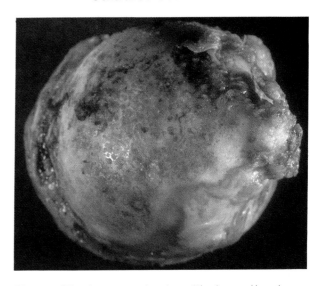

Figure 1.35   Gross superior view of the femoral head seen in Figure 1.34 shows polished or eburnated bone over the entire femoral head. Osteophytes can be noted along the margin of the joint surface.

PATHOGENESIS

Those areas of the articular cartilage that are subject to less loading and less use are generally chondromalacic. These changes are universally present and may occur without the clinical manifestation of progressive osteoarthritis. This type of chondromalacia can be observed at the rim of the radial head (Fig. 1.36), at the perifoveal and inferomedial aspects of the femoral head, and on the exposed portions of the tibial plateau (Fig. 1.37). In these age-related areas of chondromalacia, the collagen fibrils begin to break apart, resulting in further loss of ground substance and subsequent spread of the destructive process to healthy areas of cartilage. It should be pointed out that progressive osteoarthritis is probably more commonly found in those joints showing the most age-related changes (Fig. 1.38).

Currently, osteoarthritis is believed to evolve from physical stresses which injure the chondrocytes, leading to the release of enzymes and subsequent matrix breakdown.

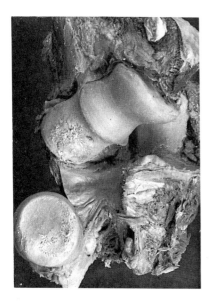
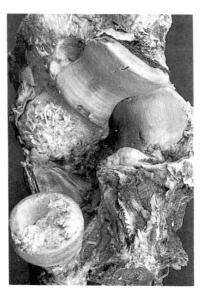
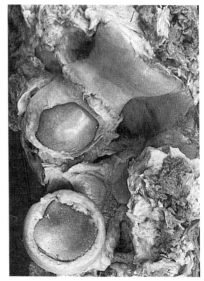

Figure 1.36 This sequence of gross specimens shows the age-related changes in a radiohumeral joint. In a patient age 45 (*left*), there is mild irregularity and fibrillation of the radiocapulum joint. At age 65 (*center*), more severe fibrillation can be noted over the articulation. Finally, at age 80 (*right*), there is a marked loss of cartilage and frank eburnation of the underlying bone.

However, it is possible that the physical stresses initially damage the collagen meshwork rather than the chondrocytes and allow degradation from synovial fluid enzymes.

Collagen synthesis in osteoarthritic joints is actually greater than in normal joints, and it increases with the severity of the disease. In those areas where cartilage has been destroyed, repair results in the growth of tufts of cartilage on top of the subchondral bone. These tufts may spread over the bony surface to form a new cartilage covering (see Fig. 1.25, *left*). This cartilage is composed of collagen arcades similar to those seen in normal cartilage; however, it contains less proteoglycan, and the collagen in type I rather than type II.

The cardinal biochemical feature of osteoarthritis appears to be a decrease of proteoglycan in the articular cartilage matrix, due either to degradation or loss from the cartilage. Proteoglycan synthesis by the cells actually *increases* in early osteoarthritis and continues to increase in proportion to the severity of the disease until the disease is so far advanced that the chondrocytes "fail" and matrix production ceases.

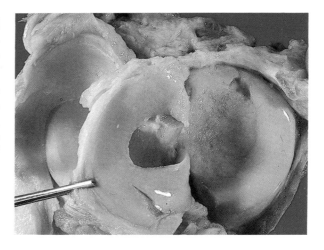

Figure 1.37 Gross superior view of the tibial plateau of a clinically normal joint with the medial meniscus reflected shows characteristic changes on the articular cartilage; namely, preservation of the cartilage under the meniscus (i.e., weight-bearing cartilage), and fibrillation and discoloration of the relatively non-weight-bearing cartilage in the medial portion of the articulation.

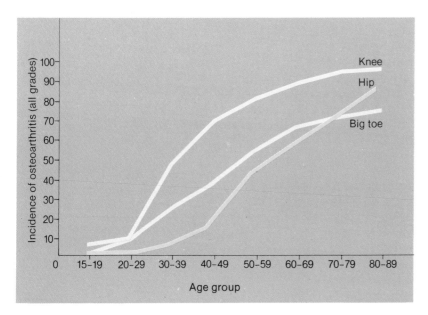

Figure 1.38 Incidence of osteoarthritis in the knee, hip, and big toe of patients from different age groups. (Modified from Heine, 1926)

Not only is there an alteration in the amount of proteoglycan, but the aggregates become smaller than in normal cartilage. There is a decrease in the chondroitin sulfate side-chain length, and a change in the relative proportion of the polysaccharides. Newly formed proteoglycan molecules in patients with osteoarthritis have increased ratios of chondroitin sulfate to keratan sulfate, and of chondroitin 4 sulfate to chondroitin 6 sulfate. Metabolic studies have shown that the pattern of synthesis of keratan sulfate, chondroitin 4 sulfate, and chondroitin 6 sulfate is the same in osteoarthritic cartilage as in normal cartilage. This finding suggests that the altered proteoglycan composition of osteoarthritic cartilage results from altered enzymatic degradation, with cleavage of fragments containing more keratan sulfate than chondroitin 4 sulfate. The ultimate result is a less resilient proteoglycan molecule and, consequently, a loss of resilience of the articular cartilage.

Etiologic Factors in Osteoarthritis

Clinically, the disease can be categorized into primary or secondary forms. In the secondary form, a direct cause for cartilage degeneration — usually structural, inflammatory, or metabolic — can be identified. In primary osteoarthritis, the cause is unknown, reflecting our current limited knowledge of the disease. Several multifactorial genetic and environmental factors, specifically the aging process and normal wear and tear, have been consistently implicated as etiologic factors.

Age

The aging process is most often implicated as the predominant contribution to the development of osteoarthritis. Radiographic surveys of hands and feet have demonstrated a 4 percent incidence of osteoarthritis at age 20 which rises to over 85 percent by age 70 (Fig. 1.39), but clinical manifestations do not occur as frequently as radiologic disease. Similar observations have been made for the knee, the hip, the shoulder, and the elbow. This increased prevalence with age is most striking in patients with moderate to severe osteoarthritis, but a similar pattern is also observed in individuals with mild osteoarthritis. Studies have found that this age-related increase in prevalence is not affected by sex, race, or regional considerations.

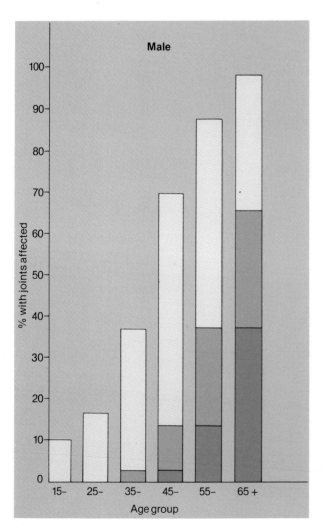
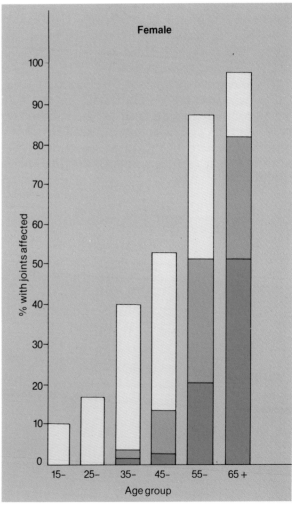

Figure 1.39   Prevalence of osteoarthritis by age group and number of joints affected. ( ) 1 +, ( ) 3 +, ( ) 5 + (From Lawrence et al., 1966)

Indeed, there are a variety of age-related changes which occur in articular cartilage. It has been reported that there are subtle changes in joint geometry which occur with age, and that these changes result in greater congruity of the articulating surfaces. It has been said that age-related changes occur initially in unloaded parts of the joint and do not necessarily lead to progressive osteoarthritis. However, increased congruity will both interfere with cartilage nutrition and alter the distribution of the load, so that formerly unloaded cartilage may come under considerable stress, leading ultimately to more generalized cartilage breakdown.

Physiologic incongruence of the articulating surfaces is probably maintained through an active remodeling process at the osteochondral junction, and histologic studies have been reported to demonstrate alterations in the rate of remodeling as a factor of age and loading of the joint (Fig. 1.40).

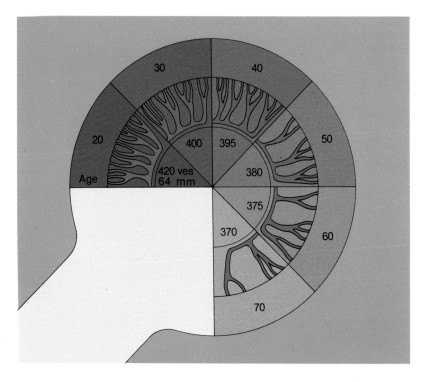

Figure 1.40 Schematic diagram demonstrates the decrease in the number of blood vessels per unit area of the femoral head with age. Since blood vessels are involved in endochondral ossification and remodeling, the age-related effect on remodeling can be appreciated. (Modified from Lane et al., 1977)

Following cessation of growth and development, articular cartilage exhibits a relatively constant biochemical composition. There is a decline in the concentration of mucopolysaccharides in patients over 80 years of age, the decrease primarily in chondroitin sulfate. Water content decreases somewhat with advancing age, perhaps relative to the reduced level of chondroitin sulfate. In studies of femoral head cartilage, proteoglycans demonstrated altered aggregating capacity which, taken together with a decreased water content, might account for a compromise in the physical properties of the cartilage.

It has also been shown that the ability of articular cartilage to withstand fatigue testing diminishes progressively with age. The superficial fibrous network appears prone to accelerated "fatigue failure" under repeated stress, a fact that does not correlate with the amount of collagen present. However, it is still not clear whether "aging" of cartilage merely represents the accumulation with time of progressive mechanical and physical insults to the articular cartilage.

Heredity

Genetic influences may contribute to the development of osteoarthritis through systemic metabolic influences, as is found in ochronosis, chondrocalcinosis, or hemochromatosis. In primary osteoarthritis, the influence of genetic factors is complex and difficult to disassociate from factors such as sex, race, and obesity.

Sex

In general, osteoarthritis tends to become more widespread in women, with moderate to severe disease showing a marked predilection for those over age 55 (Fig. 1.41). The typical patient will usually present with generalized osteoarthritis involving five or more joints, and demonstrate inflammatory episodes with elevated sedimentation rates. Evidence suggests that while women appear to be more susceptible to osteoarthritis, they may be

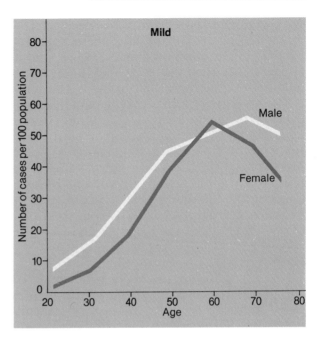

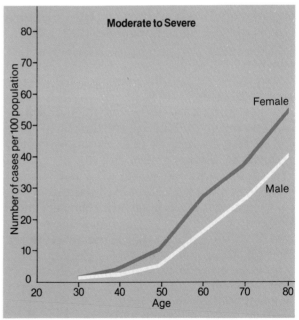

Figure 1.41   These graphs show that while prevalence of mild osteoarthritis increases comparatively with age in both men and women (*top*), the prevalence of moderate to severe osteoarthritis shows a marked increase in women over age 55 (*bottom*). (From the U.S. Public Health Service Bulletin, June 1966)

somewhat spared until after menopause. The influence of sex hormones on joint components is less marked than on bones, and it appears that their role is probably only as a modifier of other genetic factors.

The pattern of joint involvement also appears to be gender-related. Under age 35, the most frequent site of osteoarthritis in both sexes is the first metatarsophalangeal joint. Men demonstrate an age-related increase in osteoarthritis of the hip. In women, involvement of the distal interphalangeal joint, first carpometacarpal joint, and the knee joint increases rapidly between ages 45 and 55.

Race

There are differences in the prevalence of osteoarthritis between racial groups, especially with regard to the pattern of joint involvement. Osteoarthritis is found with equal frequency among whites and blacks up to age 65; thereafter, osteoarthritis occurs more frequently in the white population (Fig. 1.42).

Obesity

Excessive body weight increases the load on weight-bearing joints, and may also cause changes in posture and gait which can alter joint biomechanics. Obesity has been associated with an increase in symptomatic osteoarthritis of the knee although not of the hip. The majority of obese patients exhibit varus knee deformities, presumably brought on by a compensatory attempt to bring the feet under the center of gravity. Load is thus concentrated on the cartilage of the medial compartment, leading to degenerative changes.

Evidence suggests that there is no association between obesity and the development of Heberden's nodes or osteoarthritis of the hands or feet. In studies of osteoarthritis of the hip in obese mice, the occurrence of arthritis could be separated from obesity, suggesting that hereditary factors rather than obesity account for the disease.

Mechanical or Traumatic Factors

Sclerotic changes in the subchondral bone, produced by accumulated microtrauma, may affect the ability of articular cartilage to withstand the stress of joint loading and may lead to cartilage degeneration. In contrast, osteoporosis appears to protect the articular cartilage of the joint surfaces.

Many types of mechanical stress have been implicated as predisposing to osteoarthritis, including a single major impact, repeated minor impacts, and protracted overuse (e.g., in

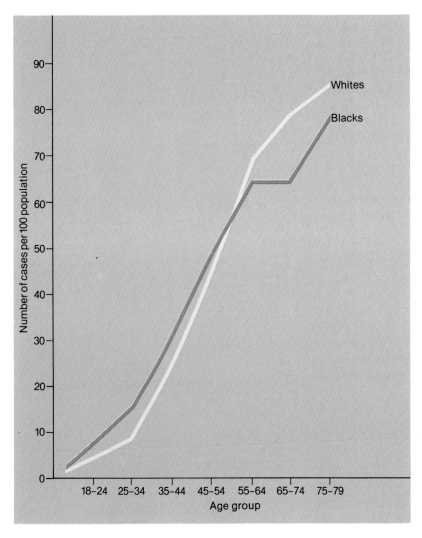

Figure 1.42 Increased prevalence of all grades of osteoarthritis in whites as compared to blacks. (From the U.S. Public Health Service Bulletin, June 1966)

athletes). In addition, structural defects in the joint such as excessive congruence, joint dysplasias, and hypermobility may exacerbate the effects of trauma by leading to excessive load bearing. Although a single major impact has been found to lead to osteoarthritis, most cases appear following protracted overloading. This probably accounts for the high frequency of osteoarthritis found in the shoulders and elbows of pneumatic drill operators, in the ankles of ballet dancers, in the elbows of baseball pitchers, and in the acromioclavicular joints of weightlifters.

The major factors which attenuate a load delivered to a joint appear to be joint motion, and the associated lengthening of muscles under tension and deformation of the subchondral bone under load. Seemingly minor but unanticipated impulse loading such as slipping on a stair may be a major factor in primary joint degeneration. Unexpected falls of only 1 inch allow insufficient time to bring protective reflexes to play and are thus associated with transmission of excessive loads to articular cartilage. Factors which lead to muscle fatigue also tend to impair the shock-absorbing mechanism and contribute to the development of cartilage damage.

Summary
By the time a pathologist gets to examine a joint with arthritis, it is likely that all of the various components of the joint will be involved: bone, cartilage, synovium, and periarticular structures. Histologic examination of these tissues will show evidence of both injury and repair. It may be, and usually is, extremely difficult from examination of advanced cases to determine what the initial joint insult was.

In many cases of osteoarthritis, etiology is apparent and the disease is clearly secondary. On the other hand, the etiology of idiopathic senile osteoarthritis is multifactorial, with both genetic and environmental factors influencing the development, the pattern of joint involvement, and the severity of the condition. The role of repeated impacts with microtrauma and of subtle alterations in the architecture and congruence of the joint seems well-established. However, whether these physical factors result in degenerative changes by a direct effect on the chondrocytes or by leading to fatigue failure in the aging collagen network is still unknown.

2
Clinical, Radiologic, and Differential Diagnosis of Osteoarthritis

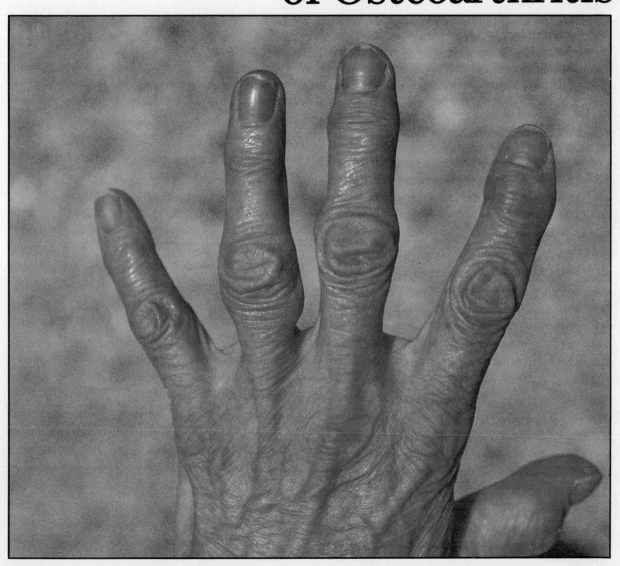

In this chapter, the clinical presentation, physical signs, radiologic appearance, and laboratory findings in patients with osteoarthritis will be discussed. In addition, the differential diagnosis of osteoarthritis, with particular reference to its secondary forms, will be considered.

CLINICAL FEATURES

While the symptoms of osteoarthritis depend largely on which joint or joints are involved, the chief complaints tend to be deformity, mild aching pain associated with movement, and limitation of motion. Stiffness after periods of rest may also occur but usually lasts less than 15 to 30 minutes. Occasionally, pain may be constant and persist even at rest. Some patients may complain of aching pain which awakens them at night. In some instances, pain may be felt at a distance from the involved joint. In osteoarthritis of the hip, "referred" pain may be felt in the region of the knee; in cervical spine osteoarthritis, in the shoulder or arm; and in lumbar spine osteoarthritis, in the lumbar muscles, buttock, or legs.

Symptoms of osteoarthritis are generally confined to one or two joints. In cases where multiple joints are involved, the pattern of joint involvement may be helpful in differentiating osteoarthritis from other forms of arthritis. Clinically, the joints involved by osteoarthritis, in relative order of frequency, are as follows: the distal interphalangeal joint, the first metatarsophalangeal joint, the knee, the proximal interphalangeal joint, the hip, the first metacarpophalangeal joint, the lumbar spine, and the cervical spine (Fig. 2.1). Other joints such as the temporomandibular, the sternoclavicular, and the shoulder joints are much less commonly involved. The disease is limited to these joints and their immediately surrounding structures; there are no systemic manifestations. In contrast, rheumatoid arthritis most frequently affects the proximal interphalangeal, the metacarpophalangeal, and the wrist (or carpal) joints; the elbows,

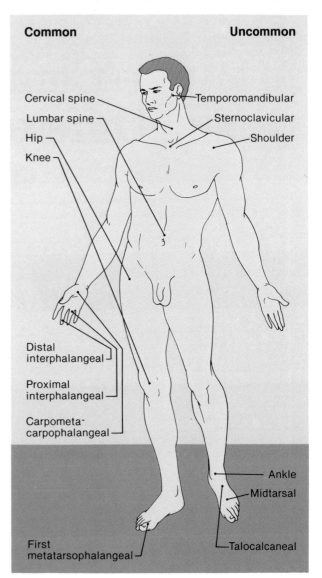

Figure 2.1 Pattern of joint involvement in osteoarthritis. Clinically, the most commonly involved joints are labeled on the left, and the less commonly involved joints are labeled on the right.

shoulders, hips, and knees are also frequently involved.

The most common physical finding in osteoarthritis is tenderness localized in the specifically involved joint. However, pain may occur on passive movement of the joint even in the absence of local tenderness. Fine crepitus, the sensation of grating or crackling, occurs on both active and passive movement of the joint. Signs of inflammation such as redness and heat are uncommon, but effusions may occur, especially following episodes of strenuous joint use. The joint may be enlarged due to the accumulation of synovial fluid, capsular proliferation, osteophyte formation, or a combination of all three.

Bony proliferation and osteophyte formation at the distal interphalangeal joints may produce the characteristic Heberden's nodes (Fig. 2.2) or, at the proximal interphalangeal joints, Bouchard's nodes (Fig. 2.3). Late in the disease there may be changes in the shape of the joint, malalignment, marked limitation of motion, instability of the joint, and spasm or atrophy of the surrounding muscles.

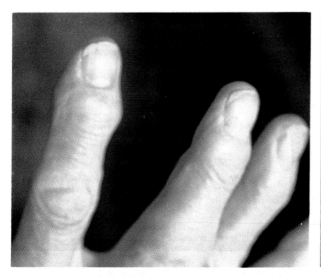

Figure 2.2 The irregular, bony, asymmetrical prominence at the distal interphalangeal joint shown in this photograph represents a Heberden's node.

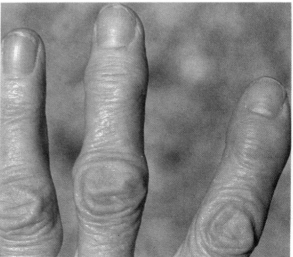

Figure 2.3 The irregular, bony prominence at the proximal interphalangeal joint shown in this photograph represents a Bouchard's node.

RADIOLOGIC FEATURES

In general, the radiologic findings of osteoarthritis are similar and independent of the particular joint involved, yet each of the commonly involved joints may show characteris-

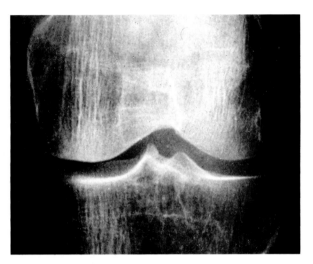
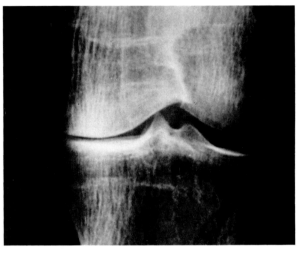

Figure 2.4 Radiograph of the knee of an osteoarthritic patient, taken with the patient in a supine position (*left*), demonstrates an apparently normal joint space with slight subchondral bony sclerosis. However, another radiograph of this same knee, this time taken with the patient standing (*right*), reveals severe joint space narrowing, a manifestation of osteoarthritis which only becomes apparent when the joint is subjected to weight bearing. (From Insall, 1983)

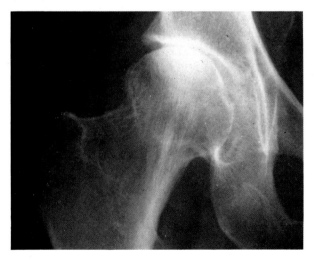
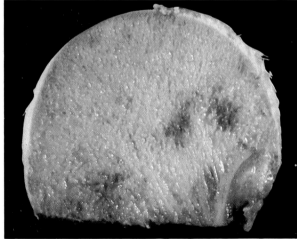

Figure 2.5 Radiograph of the hip (*left*) shows narrowing of the superior compartment, with relative preservation of the medial compartment. A gross sagittal section of this hip (*right*) demonstrates loss of cartilage over part of the femoral head surface.

tic radiologic features. Early in the disease process there may be apparent widening of the joint space, probably related to synovial effusion. In interpreting the radiologic joint space, it is important to realize that it may appear to be normal despite severe cartilage degeneration and, furthermore, that radiographs of non-weight-bearing joints may not show the full extent of the disease (Fig. 2.4).

Nonuniform joint space narrowing usually follows the degeneration and disappearance of hyaline cartilage (Fig. 2.5). Subchondral bony sclerosis or eburnation is quite characteristic, and represents deposition of new bone (Fig. 2.6).

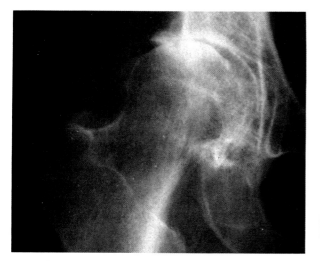

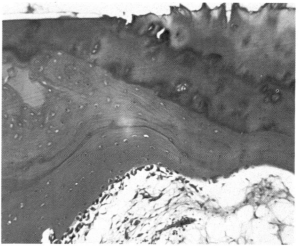

Figure 2.6   Radiograph of the hip (*left*) shows marked subchondral bony sclerosis as areas of increased bone density in both the femoral head and the acetabulum. A photomicrograph of the joint surface (*right*) shows extensive subchondral sclerosis and new bone formation (eburnation).

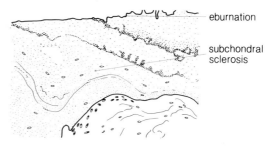

Marginal osteophytes in a variety of patterns reflect bone and cartilage proliferation (Fig. 2.7). Ligamentous calcification may be seen in the periarticular area. Subchondral cysts, usually with a rim of dense bone, may be evident (Fig. 2.8), measuring millimeters to several centimeters in diameter. Subluxation and gross deformity accompanied by the formation of loose bodies in the joint are late radiologic findings (Fig. 2.9). Bony ankylosis is rare, though occasionally bridging osteophytes may be seen in the spine (Fig. 2.10).

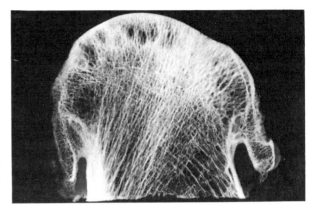

Figure 2.7 Radiograph of an excised femoral head shows osteophyte formation at the joint margin. Cystic lucencies just below the superior surface of the femoral head represent subchondral cysts.

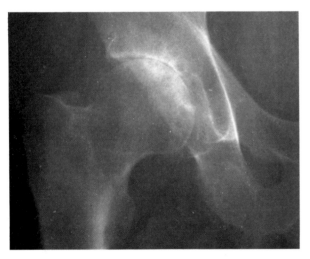

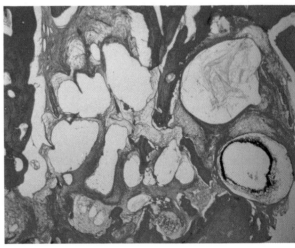

Figure 2.8 Radiograph of the hip (*left*) shows marked joint space narrowing, with many cystic lucencies in the femoral head and acetabulum. Radiodense bone can be seen surrounding the cysts. A low-power photomicrograph of a subchondral cyst (*right*) demonstrates its fibrous wall filled with a viscous fluid.

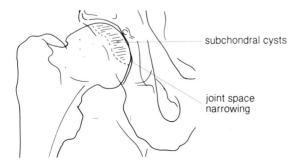

subchondral cysts

joint space narrowing

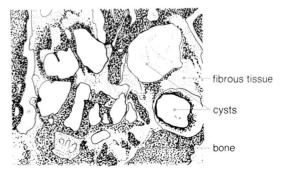

fibrous tissue

cysts

bone

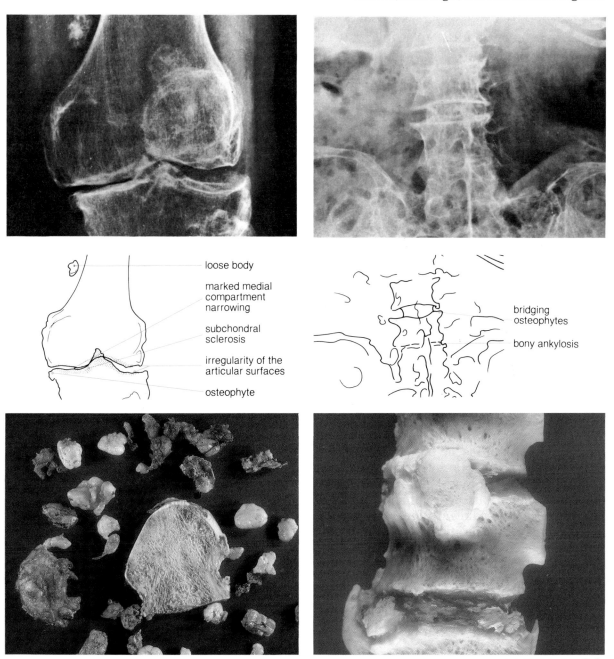

loose body

marked medial
compartment
narrowing

subchondral
sclerosis

irregularity of the
articular surfaces

osteophyte

bridging
osteophytes

bony ankylosis

Figure 2.9   Radiograph of the knee (*top*) shows extensive subchondral sclerosis, and irregularity of all the articular surfaces. Also note the large loose body in the suprapatellar bursa. Gross pathologic specimens of a surgically excised hip (*bottom*) reveal loose bodies which were removed along with the fomoral head in a patient with osteoarthritis.

Figure 2.10   Radiograph of the lumbar spine (*top*) shows bridging osteophytes, with bony ankylosis of the adjacent vertebrae. A pathologic view of this spine (*bottom*) actually demonstrates the bony outgrowths bridging between the vertebrae.

In summary, the radiologic criteria for the diagnosis of osteoarthritis are as follows:

1. Narrowing of the joint space associated with sclerosis of the subchondral bone
2. Altered shape of bone ends
3. Cystic areas with sclerotic walls situated in the subchondral bone
4. Formation of osteophytes at the joint margins or at ligamentous attachments
5. Periarticular calcification
6. Malalignment

With any two of these radiologic findings, the diagnosis of minimal osteoarthritis would be appropriate; with three, moderate osteoarthritis; and with four, severe osteoarthritis.

There is often a disparity between radiologic evidence of structural disease and clinical symptoms. This is borne out by the fact that more than 85 percent of the population over age 70 have radiographic osteoarthritis in weight-bearing joints, but relatively few report symptoms (Fig. 2.11).

LABORATORY FINDINGS

Laboratory studies to date have found no specific abnormalities in patients with primary osteoarthritis. However, in generalized osteoarthritis there may be transient minor elevations of various acute-phase reactants (i.e., erythrocyte sedimentation rate, C-reactive protein, etc.). Specific laboratory studies may be needed for diagnosis of secondary forms of osteoarthritis associated with specific primary diseases such as ochronosis, gout, chondrocalcinosis, or hemochromatosis.

Examination of the synovial fluid serves primarily to rule out inflammatory or metabolic

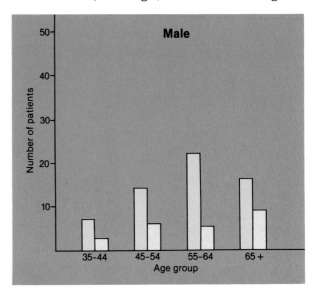

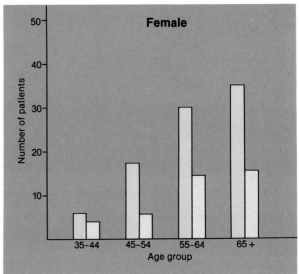

Figure 2.11 Relationship between radiologic evidence of osteoarthritis of the knee ▇ and clinical manifestations ▇ by age group. (Modified from Lawrence et al., 1966)

diseases. In osteoarthritis, the synovial fluid is considered group I (noninflammatory): essentially normal with only a few more cells than normal joint fluid, and a normal or slightly reduced viscosity (Tables 2.1 and 2.2).

Table 2.1   Examination of Joint Fluid

	Normal	Group I (Noninflammatory)	Group II (Inflammatory)	Group III (Septic)
Clarity	Transparent	Transparent	Translucent-opaque	Opaque
Color	Clear	Yellow	Yellow to opalescent	Yellow to green
Viscosity	High	High	Low	Variable
WBCs per mm³	200	200–2000	2000–100,000	100,000
Polymorphonuclear leukocytes	25%	25%	50% or more	75% or more
Mucin clot	Firm	Firm	Friable	Friable

Table 2.2   Diseases Associated with Joint Fluid Findings

Group I	Group II	Group III
Degenerative joint disease	Rheumatoid arthritis	Bacterial infections
Trauma*	Acute crystal-induced synovitis (gout and pseudogout)	
Osteochondritis dissecans	Reiter's syndrome	
Osteochondromatosis	Ankylosing spondylitis	
Neuropathic arthropathy*	Psoriatic arthritis	
Subsiding or early inflammation	Arthritis accompanying ulcerative colitis and regional enteritis	
Hypertrophic osteoarthropathy†	Rheumatic fever†	
Pigmented villonodular synovitis*	Systemic lupus erythematosus†	
	Progressive systemic sclerosis (scleroderma)†	

*May be hemorrhagic.
†Groups I or II.

DIFFERENTIAL DIAGNOSIS

Diagnosis of osteoarthritis is based on characteristic clinical and radiologic features. As mentioned previously, radiologic evidence of osteoarthritis does not necessarily imply clinical disease, and there may be a discordance between radiologic disease and clinical symptoms, especially in the axial skeleton and in the hip. Pathologic studies have shown that carti-

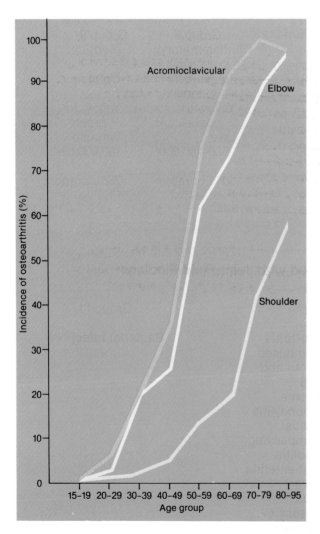

Figure 2.12   Incidence of osteoarthritis in the shoulder ▦, elbow ▦, and acromioclavicular ▦ joints, by age group. (Modified from Heine, 1926)

Table 2.3   Classification of Osteoarthritis by Causative Factors

Primary
  Idiopathic
  Primary generalized
  Erosive

Secondary
  Congenital or Developmental Defects
    Hips
      Hip dysplasias
      Shallow acetabulum
      Legg-Calvé-Perthes disease
      Slipped capital femoral epiphysis
      Primary protrusio acetabuli
    Other
      Morquio's syndrome
      Multiple epiphyseal dysplasias
      Osteochondritides
  Traumatic Defects
    Acute
    Chronic
    Charcot's arthropathy
  Avascular Necrosis of Bone (Osteonecrosis)
    Hemoglobinopathies
    Steroid therapy
  Inflammatory Disorders
    Rheumatoid arthritis
    Spondyloarthritides
    Septic arthritis
    Crystal-induced arthropathies
  Endocrine Disorders
    Acromegaly
    Diabetes mellitus
    Sex hormone abnormalities
    Hypercortisolism
    Myxedema (hypothyroidism)
  Metabolic Disorders
    Hemochromatosis
    Ochronosis
    Paget's disease
    Hyperparathyroidism

lage destruction occurs quite frequently in joints that are rarely the site of symptomatic osteoarthritis, namely the shoulder, the elbow, and the acromioclavicular joint (Fig. 2.12).

Diagnosis of primary osteoarthritis is based on elimination of all the known causes of secondary osteoarthritis (Table 2.3). However, since the pathologic as well as the radiologic findings in joint degeneration are so similar, regardless of the underlying cause, identification of the causal event or process may be difficult or impossible.

Congenital or Developmental Defects

Congenital dislocation of the hip, slipped capital femoral epiphysis, and Legg-Calvé-Perthes disease as well as other forms of unspecified hip dysplasias have been recognized as causative factors of osteoarthritis of the hip and, in the opinion of some, may account for as many as 50 percent of cases. By altering the shape of the joint components and the biomechanics of the joint, these defects may lead to progressive osteoarthritis.

Congenital dislocation of the hip (Fig. 2.13) is a relatively uncommon abnormality in which the femoral head is not properly positioned in the acetabular fossa at the time of birth. It occurs subsequent to mechanical and/or physical factors such as tight maternal abdominal and uterine musculature, breech presentation, maternal hormones such as estrogen and relaxin, or forced hip extension following birth, and leads to instability of the hip in the newborn. The left hip is more often involved, but bilateral occurrence may be observed in more than 25 percent of patients. Treatment consists of early detection and reduction, i.e., the return of the femoral head to its normal position. In persistent dislocations, the bone and the soft tissue adjacent to the joint undergo reactive changes that preclude easy reduction, and both the acetabulum and the femoral head become irregularly contoured. In untreated patients, secondary osteoarthritis develops relatively early in life.

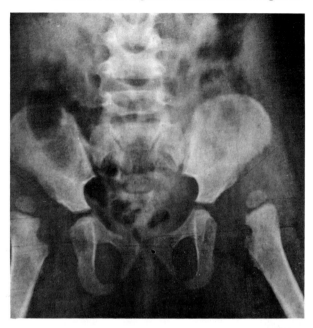

Figure 2.13 Radiograph of the hips of a 6-month-old child demonstrates bilateral congenital dislocation of the femoral head superiorly and laterally from the acetabular fossa. Note also the lack of convexity of the fossa.

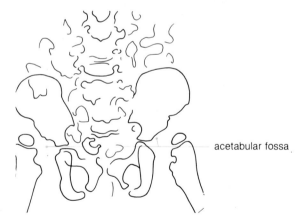

acetabular fossa

Slipped capital femoral epiphysis (adolescent coxa vara) results from spontaneous disruption of the epiphyseal plate of the hip (Fig. 2.14), which usually occurs in overweight adolescents at the time of the growth spurt (10 to 15 years of age). Depending on the magnitude of the slippage, symptoms may be variable or may not occur until late in life. Radiologically, dorsal displacement of the epiphysis may only be evident on lateral view.

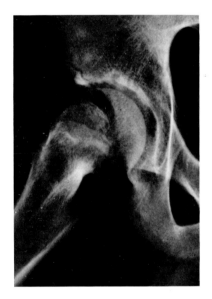

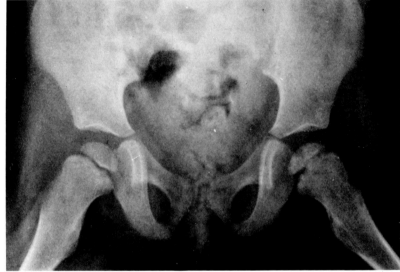

Figure 2.14 Radiograph of the hip demonstrates slipped capital femoral epiphysis, with medial displacement of the epiphysis.

Figure 2.15 Radiograph of the hips of a 6-month-old child with Legg-Calvé-Perthes disease of the left hip reveals a markedly wide joint space, with in-creased density and flattening of the secondary center of ossification, and slight irregularity on the metaphyseal side of the growth plate.

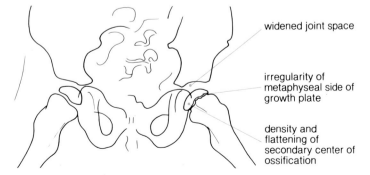

widened joint space

irregularity of metaphyseal side of growth plate

density and flattening of secondary center of ossification

Legg-Calvé-Perthes disease occurs in children —usually boys—between the ages of 5 and 9 years. The earliest radiologic sign is widening of the joint space. This appearance results from the cessation of endochondral ossification following avascular necrosis of the secondary center of ossification. Continued growth of cartilage which is not dependent on the occluded vessels of the bony epiphysis manifests as an increase in the width of the joint space (Fig. 2.15). The bony epiphysis may subsequently undergo collapse and deformation. Distortion of the femoral head may be a major factor in the subsequent development of osteoarthritis (Fig. 2.16).

In *hip dysplasia*, the acetabulum is not sufficiently developed to cover the femoral head. A progressive limp may develop in early childhood (between the ages of 2 and 5 years). In less severe cases, the onset of symptoms may not appear until the teens or even later in life, at which point the pathologic and radiologic picture will be that of osteoarthritis (Fig. 2.17).

Avascular Necrosis of Subchondral Bone
Only recently has it been appreciated that avascular necrosis of a segment of the subchondral bone (segmental infarction, osteonecrosis) is a significant cause of secondary osteoarthritis not only of the hip but also of the knee and other joints. That avascular necrosis is a systemic phenomenon is supported by the observation that multiple joint involvement occurs in 50 percent of cases. Areas of osteonecrosis immediately adjacent to an articular surface may bring about osteoarthritis through fracture of the necrotic bone and subsequent collapse of the overlying cartilage. In contrast to primary osteoarthritis, the clinical onset of avascular necrosis is usually sudden. For those patients who come to surgery, the duration of symptoms is significantly shorter than for those with either rheumatoid arthritis or primary osteoarthritis. The hip seems to be the joint most commonly affected, particularly the femoral com-

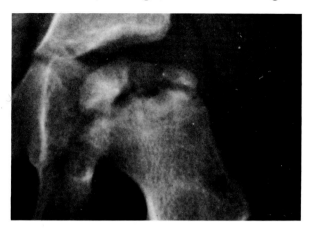

Figure 2.16 Radiograph of the hip in advanced Legg-Calvé-Perthes disease shows gross fragmentation of the secondary center of ossification, and irregularity on the metaphyseal side of the growth plate. At this stage, the joint space appears normal.

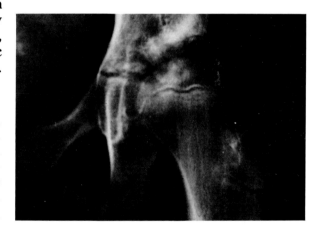

Figure 2.17 Radiograph of a patient with hip dysplasia shows flattening and mild distortion of the femoral head shelving as well as loss of convexity of the superior aspect of the acetabulum. This dysplasia may be secondary to acetabular malformation, congenital dislocation of the hip, or old, unrecognized Legg-Calvé-Perthes disease.

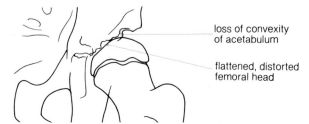

loss of convexity of acetabulum

flattened, distorted femoral head

ponent. In this regard, it is generally true that the convex surface of any joint is the one most often affected by osteonecrosis.

The radiologic features of avascular necrosis include a change in the contour of the joint and increased bone density (Fig. 2.18). The former results from failure by the reparative tissues to support the articular surface, with subsequent collapse of the infarcted area. The latter results mainly from reparative new bone, with subsequent trabecular thickening at the margin of the infarct. It should be emphasized that the necrosis involves only bone and bone marrow, and not – except in rare cases – the articular cartilage, which receives its nutrition from the synovial fluid. Therefore, on radiographs, the joint space remains intact, at least in the initial stages of the disease. This radiologic feature clearly distinguishes early avas-

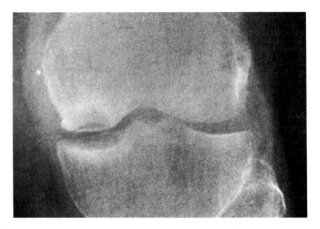

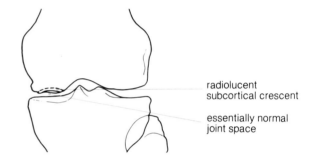

radiolucent subcortical crescent

essentially normal joint space

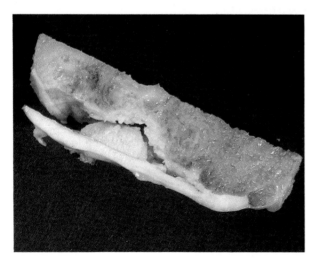

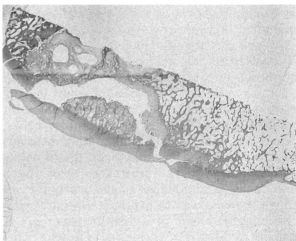

Figure 2.18 Radiograph of the knee in a patient with avascular necrosis (top right) reveals a radiolucent subcortical crescent. The joint space is essentially normal; however, flattening of the articular surface due to early collapse is evident. A gross section of the osteonecrotic area (left) shows that the necrotic bone segment (bright yellow) is attached to the articular cartilage but separated from the underlying bone by a zone of reparative scar tissue which gives rise to the radiolucency seen on the radiograph. A histologic section (bottom right) confirms the radiologic and gross presentations.

cular necrosis from other forms of joint disease in which the first radiologically evident change is a loss of articular cartilage and joint space narrowing (Fig. 2.19).

In advanced avascular necrosis, collapse of the necrotic segment and flattening of the joint surface ensue. The articular cartilage detaches from the underlying bone, which in turn gradually fragments and erodes. These changes result in the gross destruction of the joint, which ultimately shows the signs of secondary osteoarthritis (Fig. 2.20).

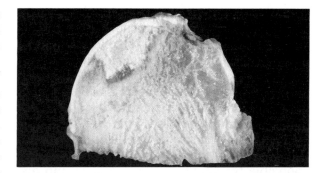

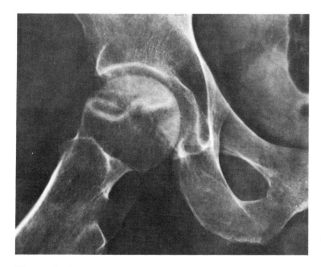

Figure 2.19 In this frog-lateral radiograph of the hip in a patient with avascular necrosis, there is evidence of collapse as demonstrated by a stepoff of the joint surface at the lateral margin. Also note a radiodense line demarcating the area of necrosis, as well as an apparent increase in density of the necrotic femoral head.

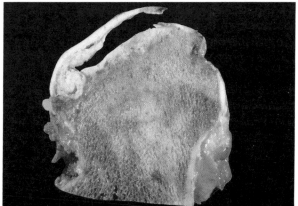

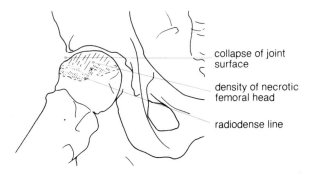

collapse of joint surface

density of necrotic femoral head

radiodense line

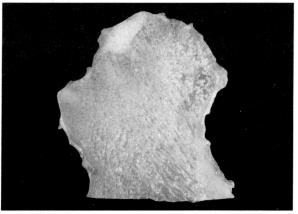

Figure 2.20 Gross sections demonstrate progressive avascular necrosis. At an early stage (top), a line of new bone formation demarcates the necrotic area with no distortion of the femoral head. Later (center), the line collapses. Although the articular cartilage has been separated from the underlying bone, it remains in place on the femoral head. Finally, in more advanced stages (bottom), the cartilage is lost and the femoral head becomes flattened, giving an appearance indistinguishable from osteoarthritis.

An infarction of the femoral head is a common complication of a subcapital fracture of the femoral neck. Following surgical reduction and internal fixation of these fractures, over 15 percent of patients develop clinical signs and symptoms of avascular necrosis. The overall frequency of avascular necrosis of the femoral head can be appreciated from the fact that, even when a fracture is excluded as an etiologic consideration, segmental infarction is responsible for about 20 percent of all hip disease requiring prosthetic replacement in some series.

When a subcapital fracture is excluded, the most frequently associated conditions in patients with avascular necrosis of the hip are systemic corticosteroid therapy and alcoholism, with changes in fat metabolism implicated as pathogenetic in both cases. Other associated conditions include Caisson's disease, Gaucher's disease, sickle cell anemia, and systemic lupus erythematosus.

The clinical course is similar whether the osteonecrosis is idiopathic or associated with some underlying condition. Symptoms of low-

Table 2.4   Endocrine Diseases Associated with Osteoarthritis

Disease	Characteristic Radiologic Features	Diagnostic Features
Hypothyroidism and myxedema	None	Decreased thyroid hormone Increased thyroid-stimulating hormone
Obesity	Knee arthritis	
Acromegaly	Exaggerated distal phalangeal tufts	Elevated growth hormone
Hyperparathyroidism	Subperiosteal resorption Subchondral cysts	Hypercalcemia Elevated parathyroid hormone
Diabetes mellitus	Charcot's joints	Glucose intolerance

grade intermittent pain in the hip may precede radiologic changes by as much as 2 years. However, even in the absence of radiologic changes, radioisotope bone scans will reveal a marked increase in radiotracer uptake, reflecting the repair of necrotic bone. Once collapse of the femoral head becomes advanced, recognition of the underlying avascular necrosis may become impossible.

Endocrine and Metabolic Diseases
As shown in Tables 2.4 and 2.5, there are a variety of endocrine and metabolic diseases associated with osteoarthritis. Although patients may present a clinical picture of primary osteoarthritis, most endocrine and metabolic diseases have unique clinical and radiographic features that allow for correct diagnosis.

Hypothyroidism. This disease is associated with an increased incidence of osteoarthritis. Patients with hypothyroidism may present

Table 2.5   Metabolic Diseases Associated with Osteoarthritis

Disease	Characteristic Radiologic Features	Diagnostic Features
Chondrocalcinosis	Stippled calcification of the chondral cartilage	Calcium pyrophosphate dihydrate crystals in synovial fluid
Ochronosis	Narrowing and calcification of the intervertebral disks	Increased urinary excretion of homogentisic acid
Hemochromatosis	Narrowing of the second and third metacarpophalangeal joints	Cirrhosis, diabetes, brown skin pigmentation
Wilson's disease	Chondrocalcinosis	Cirrhosis, choreoathetosis, renal tubular disease, low levels of serum ceruloplasmin
Paget's disease	Bone and joint deformity, "window frame" vertebrae	Elevated 24-hour urinary hydroxyproline level

with myalgia, joint pain, and joint effusions, and may have radiographic evidence of osteoarthritis. However, a diagnosis of hypothyroidism should be suspected if there are clinical features such as weight gain, lethargy, and preference for warm environments. This diagnosis may then be confirmed by demonstrating low tri-iodothyronine (T3) and thyronine (T4) levels, as well as an elevated thyroid-stimulating-hormone (TSH) level.

Acromegaly. In patients suffering from acromegaly, the increase in growth hormone synthesis and the release of somatomedin from the liver result in a prolonged and excessive overgrowth of cartilage, with subsequent widening of the joint space and overall enlargement of the joint. Other manifestations include diffuse osteoporosis, proliferation of bone at the point of capsular and tendinous attachment, and irregularity of the distal phalangeal tuft with exaggeration of its projections (Fig. 2.21). Ultimately, premature degeneration causes joint space narrowing and the other characteristic changes of osteo-

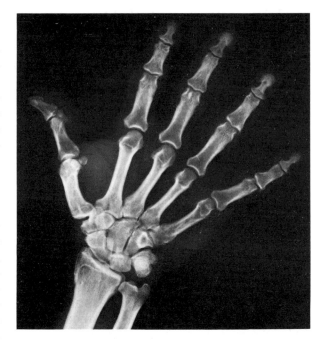

Figure 2.21   Radiograph of a hand with acromegaly reveals osteophyte formation at the distal interphalangeal joints; exuberant tufts at the distal phalanges; thickening and enlargement of the second, third, and fourth proximal phalanges; and squaring of the second and third phalanges.

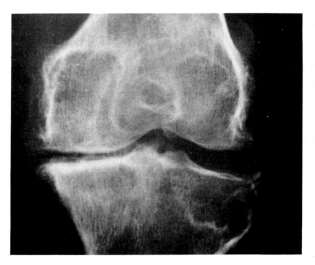

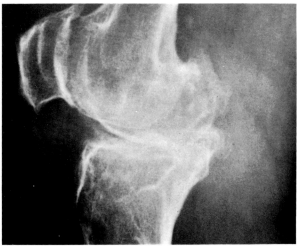

Figure 2.22   Anteroposterior (*left*) and lateral (*right*) radiographs of the knee in a patient with acromegaly. On AP view one can note a widening of the lateral compartment, reflecting cartilage hyperplasia. The degenerative changes, including osteophyte formation and joint space narrowing of the medial compartment, may cause diagnostic confusion with primary osteoarthritis. However, on lateral view, extensive bone remodeling, which appears as a squaring of the patella, is evident and characteristic of acromegaly.

arthritis (Fig. 2.22). Diagnosis of acromegaly should be confirmed by demonstrating an elevated basal growth hormone level (by radioimmunoassay) and by observing a failure to normally suppress the production of growth hormone in response to an infusion of glucose.

Hyperparathyroidism. Although nonuniform joint space narrowing may be seen radiographically in patients with hyperparathyroidism, the causal relationship between hyperparathyroidism and osteoarthritis has not been established. The most characteristic radiographic appearance of hyperparathyroidism is subperiosteal resorption, which is more apparent on the radial side of the phalanges (Fig. 2.23). Diagnosis is confirmed by demonstrating hypercalcemia, hypophosphatemia, and/or elevated parathormone levels. Subchondral erosions and chondrocalcinosis involving the triangular cartilage between the ulna and the base of the greater multangular bone may occur but are not diagnostic of hyperparathyroidism since they are also present in many metabolic diseases (e.g., hemochromatosis and Wilson's disease).

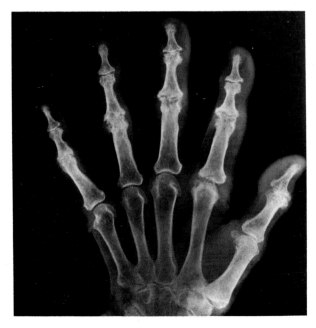

Figure 2.23 Radiograph of the hand shows marked joint space narrowing, extensive osteophyte formation, and cystic changes in all proximal interphalangeal joints and in the third and fourth distal interphalangeal joints. Resorption can be observed in the tufts of the distal phalanges.

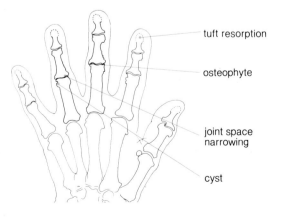

Diabetes Mellitus. In diabetes mellitus, peripheral neuropathies may lead to loss of proprioception and/or pain sensation, with relaxation of supporting structures resulting in chronic instability and subluxation of the joint (Fig. 2.24). Destructive changes result in erosions, marginal joint space narrowing, and hypertrophic bone proliferation as well as multiple osteochondral loose bodies within the joint cavity. Neuropathic joint disease (Charcot's joint) may also be associated with tabes dorsalis (Fig. 2.25), leprosy, or syringomyelia.

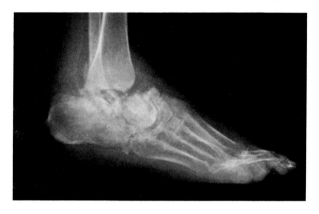

Figure 2.24 Lateral radiograph of the foot in a patient with diabetes mellitus reveals complete dissolution and fragmentation of the calcaneus, with bony fragments apparent within the joint space.

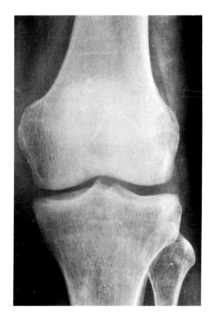 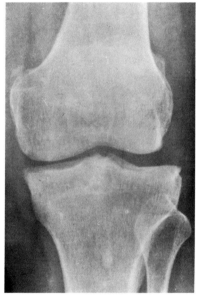 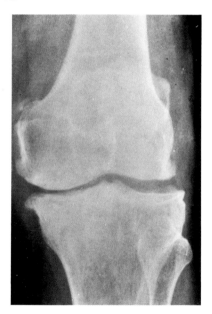

Figure 2.25 Sequential radiographs of the knee over a 3-year period reveal the early development of Charcot's joint associated with tabes dorsalis. At left is an anteroposterior view of a normal knee in a patient who complained of knee pain. One year later (*center*), joint space narrowing and some irregularity in the medial margin of the tibial articular surface are evident. Finally, 3 years later (*right*) one can observe marked joint space narrowing, effusion, multiple osteophytes, and bone fragments in the soft tissue.

Chondrocalcinosis. This disease is characterized by the intrasynovial and intra-articular deposition of calcium pyrophosphate dihydrate crystals, and may be associated with other metabolic as well as endocrine diseases. It occurs sporadically, with the predominant age of onset in the sixth or seventh decade.

The knees are the most commonly affected joints, though about 50 percent of patients show progressive degeneration in multiple joints. In mild forms, only stippled linear calcification of the meniscal and articular cartilage may be evident (Fig. 2.26). In patients with advanced disease, a destructive arthropathy may occur, with loss of bone substance,

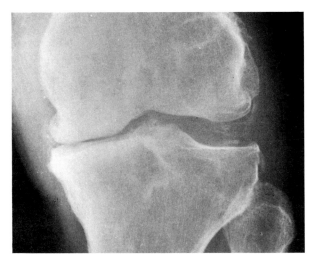

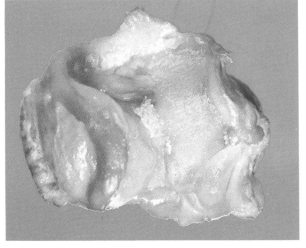

Figure 2.26   Radiograph of the knee in a patient with mild chondrocalcinosis (*left*) shows stippled calcification of the articular cartilage in the lateral compartment. In addition, joint space narrowing of the medial compartment is evident.

A gross pathologic specimen from the olecranon of the elbow (*right*) reveals opaque white streaks of calcium pyrophosphate dihydrate in the articular cartilage at the joint margin.

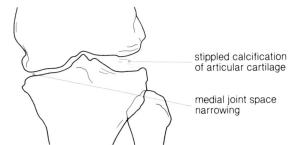

stippled calcification
of articular cartilage

medial joint space
narrowing

the appearance of large intra-articular fragments, and secondary osteoarthritis (Fig. 2.27).

There are five principal clinical presentations of chondrocalcinosis:

Type A – pseudogout
Type B – pseudo-rheumatoid-arthritis
Types C and D – pseudo-osteoarthritis
Type E – asymptomatic calcium pyrophosphate dihydrate crystal deposition as an incidental finding
Type F – pseudoneuropathic joints

Ochronosis. Ochronosis (alkaptonuria) usually becomes clinically apparent as osteo-

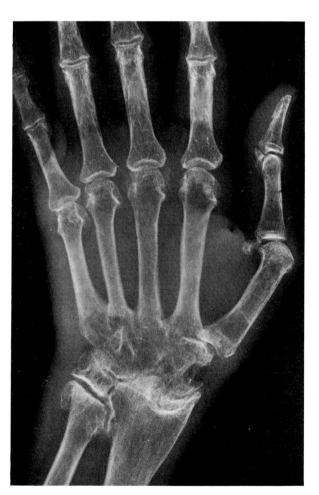

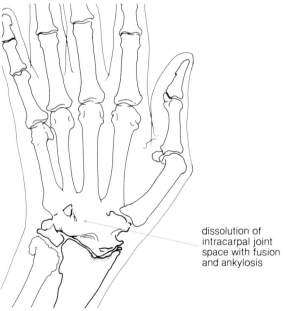

Figure 2.27   Radiograph of the hand in a patient with advanced chondrocalcinosis reveals dissolution of the intracarpal joint spaces, with fusion and ankylosis secondary to repeated episodes of inflammatory crystal-induced arthritis. The degenerative changes of osteoarthritis are also apparent at the radiocarpal and radioulnar joints.

dissolution of intracarpal joint space with fusion and ankylosis arthritis of the spine, hips, or knees in middle-aged patients. These patients lack homogentisic acid (HGA) oxidase, which results in increased urinary excretion of HGA and increased HGA binding to collagen. This abnormal binding then leads to alteration in the physical properties of the connective tissues, particularly the cartilage, skin, and sclerae (Fig. 2.28).

Hemochromatosis. This is a disorder of iron absorption and storage in which excess iron is deposited in various tissues, including the liver, skin, articular cartilage, and the synovial membrane. This deposition alters the physical characteristics of the joint tissues and predisposes to premature osteoarthritis.

Clinical symptoms and radiographic findings of osteoarthritis may precede the major clinical and laboratory findings of cirrhosis,

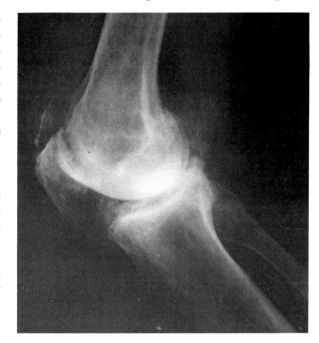

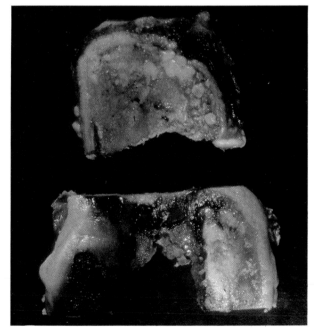

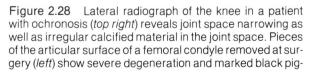

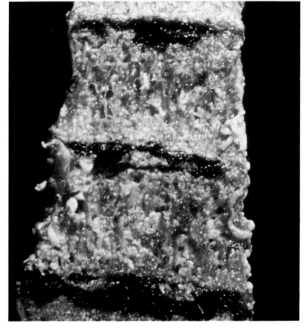

Figure 2.28   Lateral radiograph of the knee in a patient with ochronosis (*top right*) reveals joint space narrowing as well as irregular calcified material in the joint space. Pieces of the articular surface of a femoral condyle removed at surgery (*left*) show severe degeneration and marked black pigmentation of the cartilage, the characteristic appearance in ochronosis. A gross sagittal section of the lumbar spine (*bottom right*) demonstrates severe intervertebral disk narrowing, with a mahogany brown to black discoloration of the disk, also a common feature of ochronosis.

diabetes, and skin pigmentation. Affected joints reveal chondrocalcinosis, joint space narrowing, prominent osteophytes, subchondral sclerosis, and multiple lucent subchondral cysts. These findings most often present in the hand, primarily at the second and third metacarpophalangeal (MCP) joints (Fig. 2.29); however, the knees, wrists, hips, symphysis pubis, and lumbar spine may also be affected. Diagnosis of hemochromatosis may be confirmed by demonstrating a marked elevation of the plasma iron concentration with a transferrin saturation of 75 to 100 percent. The serum ferritin level will also be elevated.

Wilson's Disease. This is a condition in which copper deposition leads to cirrhosis,

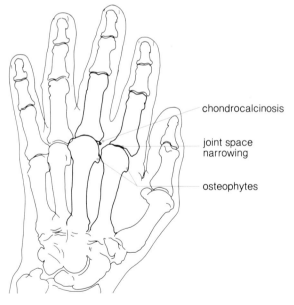

Figure 2.29 Radiograph of the hand in a patient with hemochromatosis shows prominent osteophytes at the MCP joints as well as chondrocalcinosis in the third MCP joint. The PIP and DIP joints appear normal.

chondrocalcinosis

joint space narrowing

osteophytes

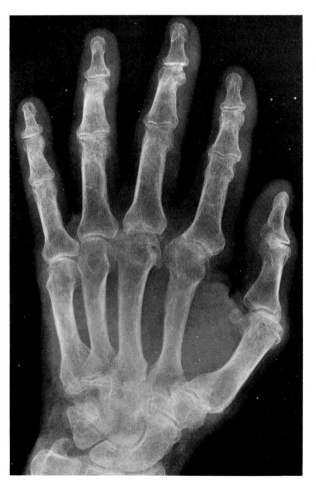

choreoathetosis, and renal tubular abnormalities. As in hemochromatosis, osteoarthritis occurs prematurely and usually involves the wrists and the MCP joints. Chondrocalcinosis may also occur, but with a lower incidence rate than that associated with hemochromatosis. Subchondral bone fragmentation, cyst formation, and subchondral sclerosis have been found in about half of all individuals with Wilson's disease, and these abnormalities may be mistaken for primary osteoarthritis (Fig. 2.30). Diagnosis can be confirmed by demonstrating Kayser-Fleischer rings on slit-lamp examination (Fig. 2.31), or by finding low levels of serum ceruloplasmin in the blood.

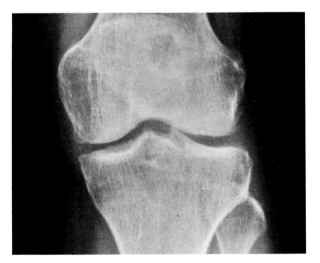

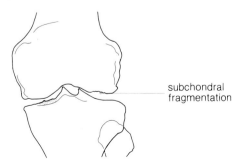

Figure 2.30   Radiograph of the knee in a patient with Wilson's disease demonstrates subchondral fragmentation and irregularity which may lead to premature osteoarthritis.

subchondral
fragmentation

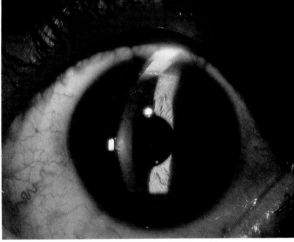

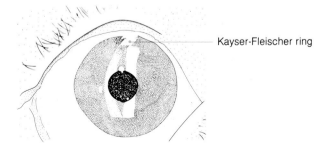

Figure 2.31   In this slit-lamp photograph, only a portion of the Kayser-Fleischer ring is seen at the periphery as a green-yellow fragment, confirming the diagnosis of Wilson's disease. (Courtesy of Dr. Fred Jacobiac)

Kayser-Fleischer ring

Inflammatory Arthritides

Diseases with major inflammatory components such as rheumatoid arthritis and gout may result in destruction and degeneration of articular cartilage. In some patients where the primary inflammatory process has become quiescent, the radiologic presentation and pathologic features may be difficult to differentiate from primary osteoarthritis. However, in the majority of cases, the history coupled with the clinical presentation will make the primary inflammatory nature of the disease apparent, thus avoiding a diagnostic dilemma.

Conclusion

In summary, the diagnosis of primary osteoarthritis requires the systematic elimination of those diseases which might contribute to the degeneration of articular cartilage. Many of the causal events that contribute to the development of osteoarthritis have only recently been recognized, and may well be obscure at the time the patient presents with pain and limitation of motion. Consequently, it might be predicted that other contributing diseases or defects may be identified to further subset those patients who are thought to have primary osteoarthritis at the present time.

3
Osteoarthritis of the Hand

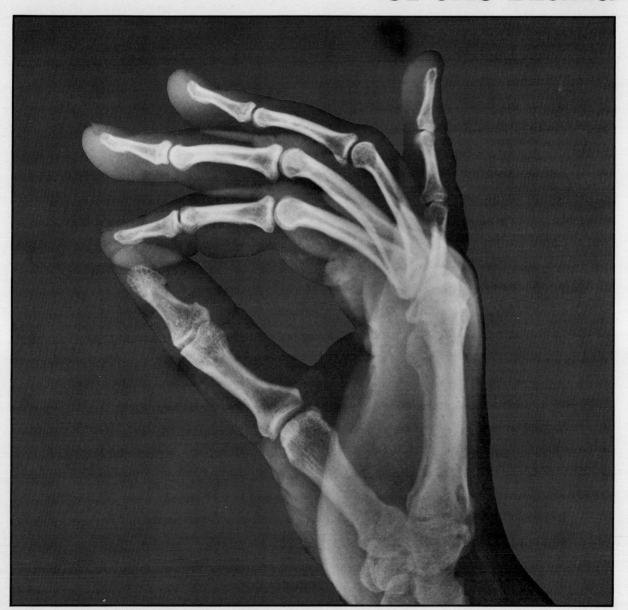

Table 3.1   Rheumatic Diseases which Affect the Hand

Disease	Affected Joint of the Hand	Clinical Manifestations
Rheumatoid Arthritis		
Adult-type	MCP	Morning stiffness
	PIP	Symmetrical fusiform swelling
	CMC	Deformity
	Carpal	Ulnar deviation
	Wrist	
Juvenile-type	MCP	Radial deviation
	PIP	Swelling of entire finger
Spondyloarthritides		
Ankylosing spondylitis	Rare	
Psoriatic arthritis	DIP	Swelling of entire finger
		"Sausage digit"
		Psoriatic nails
Reiter's disease	PIP	Conjunctivitis
		Urethritis
		Balanitis
		Keratoderma blennorrhagicum
Connective Tissue Diseases		
Systemic lupus erythematosus	MCP	Morning stiffness
	PIP	Nondeforming arthritis
	CMC	Reducible deformity
	Carpal	
Systemic sclerosis	DIP	Tight skin
	MCP	Loss of distal pulp
Polymyositis	PIP	Prominent muscle weakness
Metabolic Diseases		
Acromegaly	DIP	Symmetrical soft-tissue and
	PIP	bony enlargement
Hemochromatosis	DIP	Diabetes mellitus
	PIP	Liver disease
	MCP	
Degenerative Joint Diseases		
Primary Osteoarthritis	DIP	
	PIP	
	CMC	
Miscellaneous		
Infectious arthritis	Any	
Sarcoid arthritis	DIP	Pulmonary manifestations
	PIP	
Neoplastic arthritis	Any (rare)	

Osteoarthritis of the hand occurs primarily in middle-aged and elderly people, and is characterized by degeneration of articular cartilage, bony overgrowth of joint margins, and thickening of the synovial membrane. Although many factors contribute to the development of osteoarthritis, genetic factors appear to be of special importance in osteoarthritis of the hand. Clinical and radiologic observations assist in differentiating osteoarthritis from the other rheumatic diseases which affect the hand (Table 3.1).

ANATOMIC FEATURES

Osteoarthritis occurs in the distal interphalangeal (DIP), proximal interphalangeal (PIP), and first carpometacarpal (CMC) joints of the hands, with the former being the most common site.

In the DIP joints, slowly progressive bony enlargements (*Heberden's nodes*) are found (Fig. 3.1).

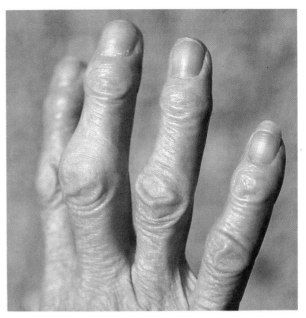

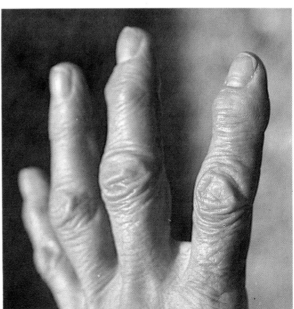

Figure 3.1 The top photograph shows lateral bony enlargement at the distal interphalangeal joint secondary to marginal osteophytes. These osteophytes are asymmetrical within the joint as well as from side to side, and they are referred to as Heberden's nodes. On dorsal projection (*bottom*), Heberden's nodes appear more prominent than on lateral projection.

These enlargements are scattered asymmetrically over the affected joint. On radiographs, bony overgrowths called *osteophytes* are also frequently demonstrated (Fig. 3.2). Occasionally, gelatinous *mucoid cysts* (Fig. 3.3) may appear in conjunction with Heberden's nodes. These cysts may be painful and tender, and appear on the dorsal surface of DIP joints. Their gelatinous substance is composed of pure hyaluronic acid with no associated protein.

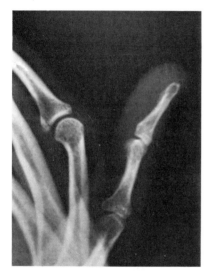 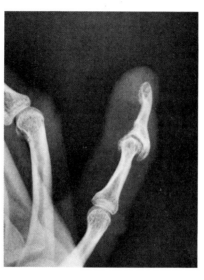 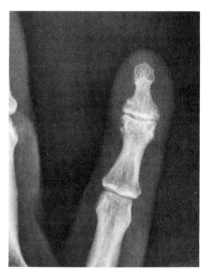

Figure 3.2 Lateral radiograph of a normal right fifth digit (*left*) shows a relatively normal DIP joint, with no osteophyte formation and a normal joint space. In contrast, a lateral radiograph of an osteoarthritic right fifth digit (*center*) shows a pronounced osteophyte on the dorsal aspect of the distal phalanx, with marked irregularity and nonuniform narrowing of the joint space. An anteroposterior view of this digit (*right*) reveals joint space narrowing, less apparent osteophyte formation, and some early subchondral sclerosis.

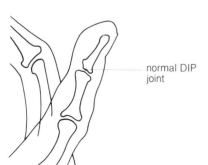 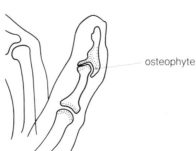 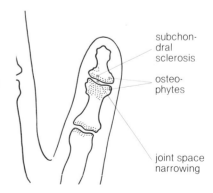

normal DIP joint

osteophyte

subchondral sclerosis

osteophytes

joint space narrowing

Similar manifestations are also found in PIP joints, except the bony enlargements are called *Bouchard's nodes* (Fig. 3.4).

In the first CMC joints, some bone deformity can be clinically observed, but a radiograph may be necessary to confirm the diagnosis (Fig. 3.5). On physical examination, there may be fine crepitus on rotation of the joint.

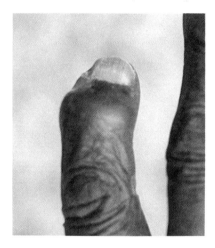
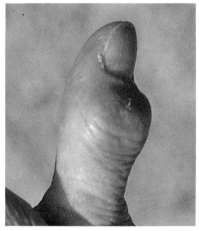
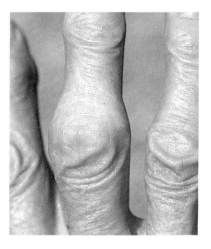

Figure 3.3   In some patients, painful distal (*left*) or proximal (*right*) interphalangeal joint enlargement may be associated with a cystic accumulation of highly polymerized hyaluronic acid.

Figure 3.4   Photograph shows bony enlargement secondary to osteophyte formation at the proximal interphalangeal joint (Bouchard's nodes).

Figure 3.5   (*Left*) Osteoarthritis of the first carpometacarpal joint may be obscure on clinical examination, or may appear as a prominence in the area of the joint just distal to the wrist. Radiograph of the wrist (*right*) confirms the diagnosis.

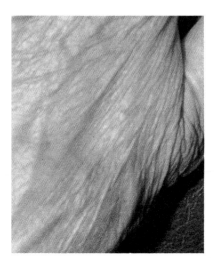
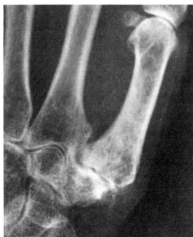
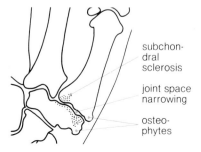

subchondral sclerosis

joint space narrowing

osteophytes

Osteoarthritis of the metacarpophalangeal (MCP) joints is rare, and is usually associated with an underlying metabolic disease, i.e., hemochromatosis, chondrocalcinosis, or hyperparathyroidism (Fig. 3.6) (see Chapter 9).

In each of the above cases, osteoarthritis develops gradually, with little or no pain. Heberden's and Bouchard's nodes may be primary or traumatic, with primary nodes most common after age 45. Heberden's nodes have been found to be genetically transmitted as a dominant trait in women and as a recessive trait in men.

Ultimately, the cartilage of the joints is destroyed, and the joints often become chronically flexed, deviated, or subluxed (Fig. 3.7).

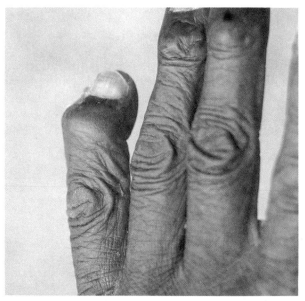

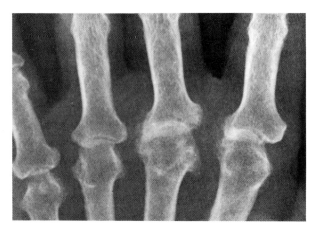

Figure 3.6　In patients with certain metabolic diseases (e.g. hemochromatosis or chondrocalcinosis), the classic symptoms of osteoarthritis may be observed radiographically in the second and third metacarpophalangeal joints, an unusual site for osteoarthritis. The fourth and fifth MCP joints appear normal.

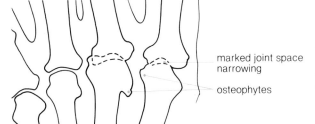

marked joint space narrowing

osteophytes

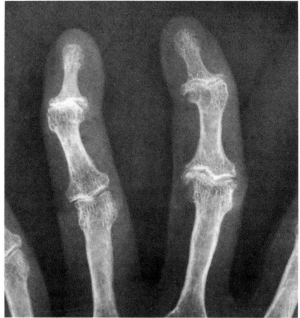

Figure 3.7　Usually, the deformity associated with osteoarthritis is minimal, with subluxation or deviation of the DIP or PIP joints. In the top photograph, the DIP joint is deviated toward the ulnar aspect. Radiograph of the hand in a patient with advanced osteoarthritis (bottom) shows a wavy deformity of the third and fourth digits secondary to osteoarthritis of the DIP and PIP joints of those digits.

Radiographically, joint space narrowing, osteophytes, and subchondral bone sclerosis may be observed (see Fig. 3.2). These deformities are relatively minor when compared to the grossly debilitating deformities associated with advanced forms of rheumatoid arthritis (Fig. 3.8).

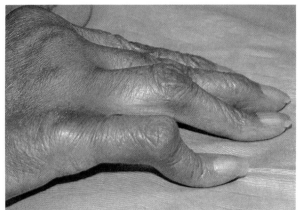

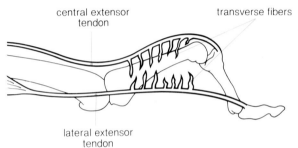

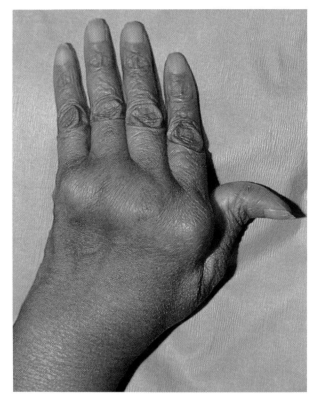

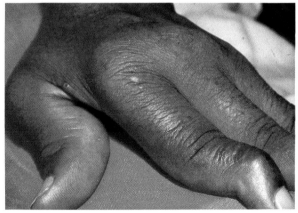

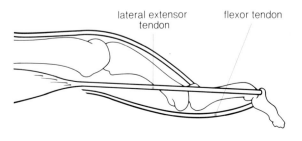

Figure 3.8 In rheumatoid arthritis, the deformity is usually distinct. (*Left*) Photograph shows swelling at the MCP joint, resulting in a lateral slippage of the extensor tendon, and ulnar deviation of the fingers. (*Top right*) Photograph shows capsular distention at the PIP joint, resulting in rupture of the transverse fibers connecting the lateral and central extensor tendons. There is flexion of the PIP joint and extension of the DIP joint (boutonniere deformity). (*Bottom right*) The long flexor tendon is responsible for initiating flexion of the DIP joint. With flexor synovitis, shown here, force is concentrated on the MCP joint. Chronic flexion of the MCP joint leads to slippage of the lateral extensor tendon, which results in flexion of the DIP joint and extension of the PIP joint (swan-neck deformity).

According to Kellgren and Lawrence, the following radiographic findings are sufficient to differentiate osteoarthritis of the hand from other rheumatic diseases which affect the region:

1. Formation of osteophytes on the joint margins
2. Periarticular ossicles (fraying of the bone around the joints)
3. Narrowing of joint cartilage associated with sclerosis of the subchondral bone (hardening of the underlying bone)
4. Small pseudocystic areas with sclerotic walls, usually situated in subchondral bone
5. Altered shape of the bone heads

PATHOLOGIC MANIFESTATIONS

In the joints of the hand, as elsewhere, osteoarthritis is characterized by the nonuniform degeneration of cartilage in diarthrodial joints (Fig. 3.9). Radiographically, this is first seen by the irregular loss of cartilage along both articulating surfaces of the joint's bones, leading to joint space narrowing (Fig. 3.10). Localized calcification at the periphery of the articular cartilage is the first step in the ultimate degeneration of the cartilage, and may precede the formation of osteophytes.

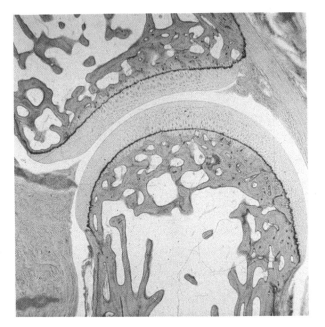

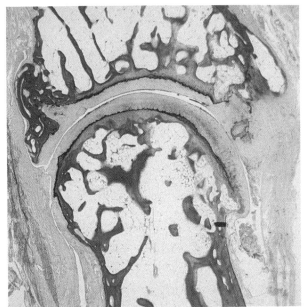

Figure 3.9 (*Top*) Photomicrograph of a DIP joint shows normal cartilage and a relatively uniform joint space. In contrast, the bottom photomicrograph shows severe, nonuniform joint space narrowing, with areas of marked cartilage degeneration. The area of intense staining beneath the cartilage represents subchondral sclerosis. (Courtesy of the Arthritis Foundation Teaching Collection)

As degeneration continues, new bone forms around the cartilage. Since the cartilage is by now diminished at its periphery, joint space narrowing continues, and osseous outgrowths (Heberden's and Bouchard's nodes) appear in the joint margins. Eburnation or sclerosis of the underlying subchondral bone usually ensues (Fig. 3.11).

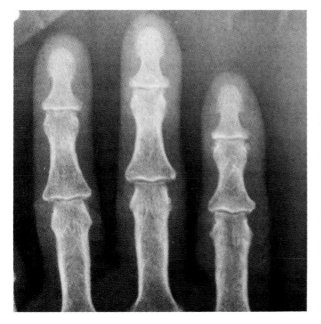

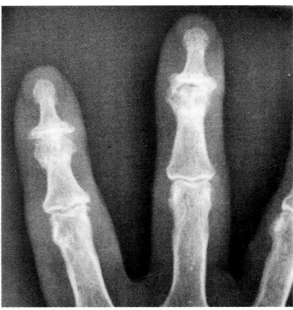

Figure 3.10   Early radiographic signs of osteoarthritis may include minimal joint space narrowing or some evidence of localized calcification at the periphery of the articular cartilage.

Figure 3.11   Radiograph of advanced osteoarthritis showing extensive osteophyte formation, marked joint space narrowing, and eburnation or sclerosis of subchondral bone.

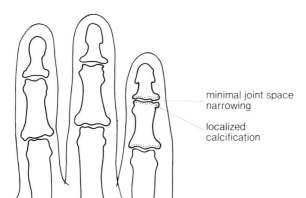

minimal joint space narrowing

localized calcification

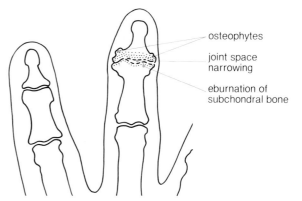

osteophytes

joint space narrowing

eburnation of subchondral bone

Following degeneration of the cartilage, synovial fluid breaks through the subchondral bone, forming large cysts (Fig. 3.12). These cysts are also found in inflammatory and metabolic arthritides. True ankylosis is rare, buy may occasionally occur in advanced osteoarthritis (Fig. 3.13).

The severity of osteoarthritis in the DIP joints can be categorized into five grades (Fig. 3.14):

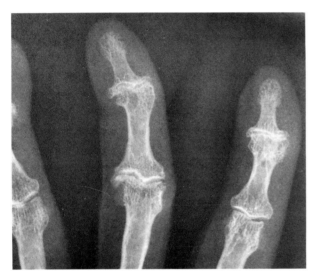

Figure 3.12   Radiograph shows a large subchondral bone cyst in addition to the other signs of advanced osteoarthritis.

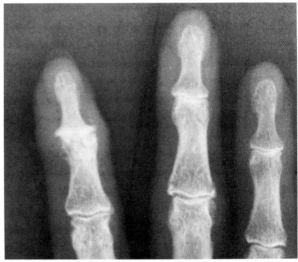

Figure 3.13   Ankylosis is rare in osteoarthritis, and is frequently difficult to evaluate on radiologic examination since there is usually some flexion deformity in addition to the marked joint space narrowing. Complete loss of motion may be necessary to confirm an apparent radiologic diagnosis.

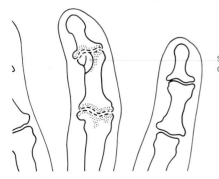

subchondral bone cyst

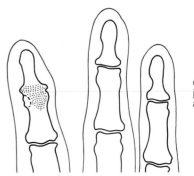

complete loss of joint space (with ankylosis)

Grade 0 (no change): joint appears normal

Grade 1 (doubtful changes): minimal joint space narrowing

Grade 2 (minimal changes): rare osteophyte formation; more noticeable joint space narrowing; periarticular sclerosis of subchondral bone

Grade 3 (moderate changes) and grade 4 (severe changes): the same changes as grade 2, but more easily delineated radiographically. Subluxation, altered bone shape, and subchondral cyst formation are also detected.

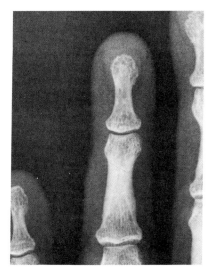 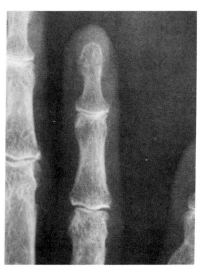 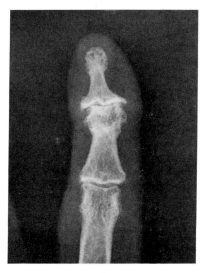

Figure 3.14   Classification of osteo-arthritis in DIP joints. (*Left*) Grade 0: Joint is essentially normal. (*Center*) Grade 2: Minimal joint space narrow-ing, rare osteophyte formation, and sclerosis may be observed. (*Right*) Grade 4: Signs of osteoarthritis can be easily delineated: extensive joint space narrowing, altered bone shape, and subluxation.

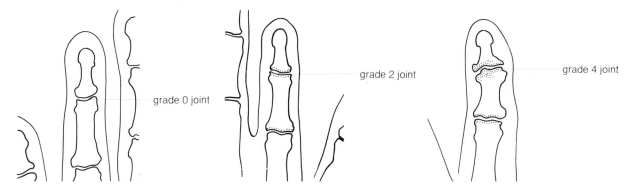

grade 0 joint

grade 2 joint

grade 4 joint

In PIP joints, the same progressive changes are detected radiographically (Fig. 3.15); similar changes also occur in CMC joints (Fig. 3.16).

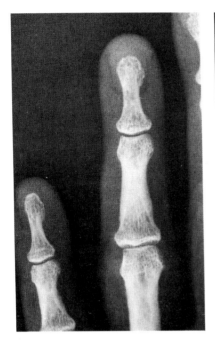 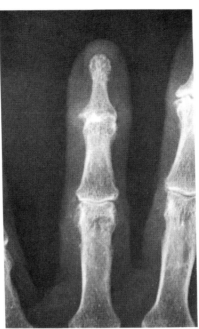 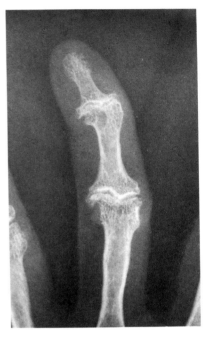

Figure 3.15 Classification of osteoarthritis in PIP joints. (*Left*) Grade 0: Joint is essentially normal. (*Center*) Grade 2: Minimal joint space narrowing, rare osteophyte formation, and sclerosis may be observed. (*Right*) Grade 4: Signs of osteoarthritis can be easily delineated: extensive joint space narrowing, altered bone shape, and subluxation.

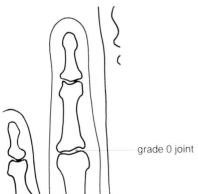 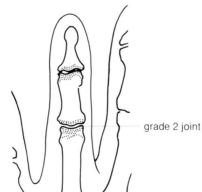 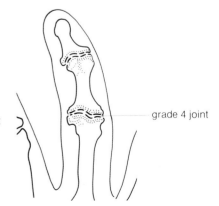

grade 0 joint

grade 2 joint

grade 4 joint

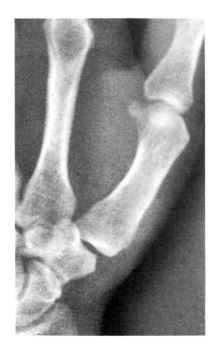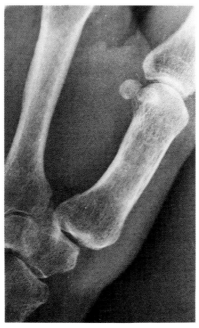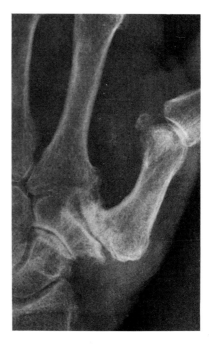

Figure 3.16   Classification of osteoarthritis in CMC joints: (*Left*) Grade 0:
Joint is essentially normal. (*Center*)
Grade 2: Minimal joint space narrowing, rare osteophyte formation, and
sclerosis may be observed. (*Right*)
Grade 4: Signs of osteoarthritis can be
easily delineated: extensive joint
space narrowing, altered bone shape,
and subluxation.

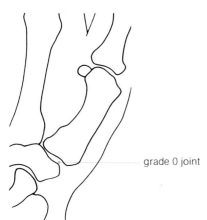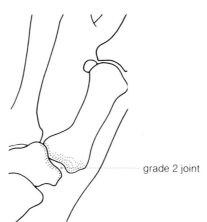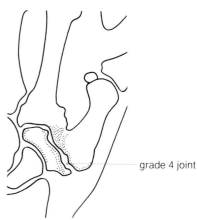

grade 0 joint   grade 2 joint   grade 4 joint

OTHER OSTEOARTHRITIDES

In addition to nodal osteoarthritis of the hand, Kellgren and Moore have described a primary, generalized form of heritable osteoarthritis which affects the DIP, PIP, and first CMC joints, as well as the scapulotrapezoid joint of the wrist, the cervical and lumbar spine, the knees, and the great toe (the first metatarsophalangeal [MTP] joint). This osteoarthritis occurs mainly in middle-aged women, and is characterized by an episodic course with subacute and acute flareups in the PIP joints. Both the PIP and DIP joints may be swollen and erythematous, suggesting an inflammatory process is taking place (Fig. 3.17).

When erosions of the articulating surfaces of bone form a major component of the pathologic and radiologic picture, the distinction is made between primary generalized osteoarthritis and erosive osteoarthritis. Although the histology of the synovia during the acute phase of erosive osteoarthritis is similar to that in rheumatoid arthritis, its pattern of distribution, the absence of systemic symptoms, negative tests for rheumatoid factor, and normal sedimentation rates should allow for correct diagnosis. Unlike rheumatoid arthritis, erosive osteoarthritis is a self-limited disease.

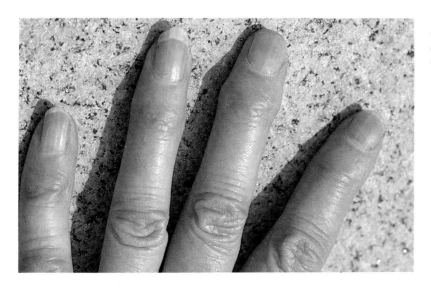

Figure 3.17   Photograph of a patient with an acute case of generalized osteoarthritis shows swelling and erthema of several DIP joints.

The hands of a woman with typical primary generalized osteoarthritis shows the classic configuration and distribution of the disease (Fig. 3.18). There is a wavy appearance to the contour of the fingers which is obvious both clinically and radiographically. The presence of irregular erosions of the articular surfaces reflects the active synovitis, and differentiates erosive from primary generalized osteoarthritis.

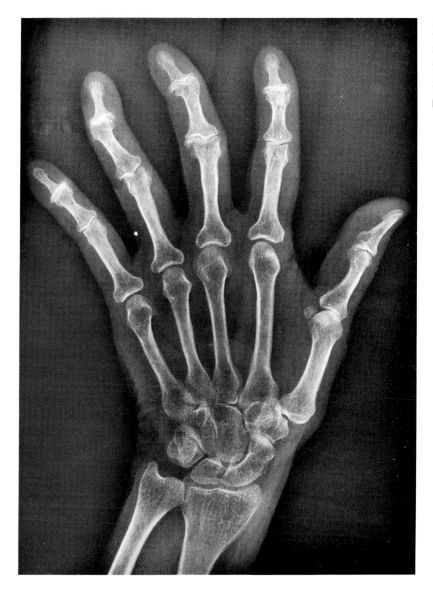

Figure 3.18　Radiograph of a patient with primary generalized osteoarthritis shows the characteristic wavy appearance of the third and fourth digits. Irregular erosions at the articular surfaces usually occur on the ulnar aspect of the joint.

4
Osteoarthritis of the Hip

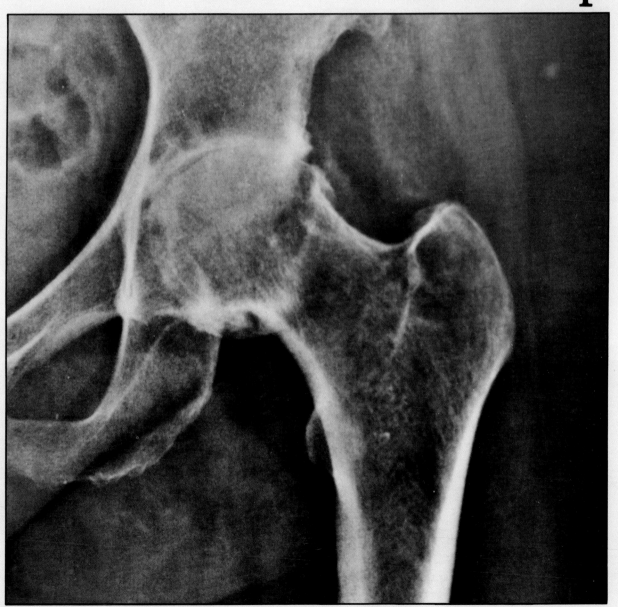

CLINICAL ASSESSMENT

Osteoarthritis of the hip is characterized by the insidious onset of pain that is aggravated by motion and relieved by rest. True hip pain is usually perceived on the outer aspect of the groin or the inner thigh. Occasionally, this pain is perceived in the knee, and is so severe that its true origin is overlooked. Severe low back pain may result from the compensatory lordosis that accompanies hip pain. Joint stiffness is common, and it increases after activity, but rarely persists for more than 15 minutes.

Several types of limp or gait abnormalities are associated with disease of the hip. When the hip is painful, the body may tilt toward the involved hip and balance on the affected side. The weight of the body is placed directly over the hip joint, decreasing the necessity for contracting the abductor muscles and producing an antalgic limp. If the abductor muscles on the side of the involved hip become weak and are unable to hold the pelvis level when weight is placed on the affected joint, dropping of the pelvis on the opposite side may occur and produce a Trendelenburg (abductor) limp. The Trendelenburg limp causes the upper part of the body to shift toward the normal hip, thereby decreasing weight-bearing responsibility on the involved side. Generally, diseases that cause pain tend to produce an antalgic limp, whereas diseases that produce an unstable hip and weakness of the abductor muscles tend to result in a Trendelenburg limp. However, both these limps may result from a wide variety of lesions, and neither can be considered characteristic of any particular disease.

Determining the patient's range of motion is invaluable in evaluating the functional integrity of the hip, since the joint is positioned too deep in the surrounding musculature to be examined as freely as the knee or elbow. Three ranges of motion are important in assessing the hip joint: flexion-extension (Fig. 4.1),

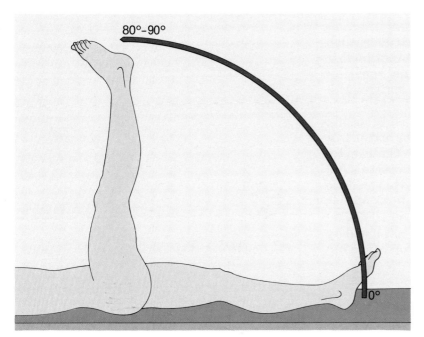

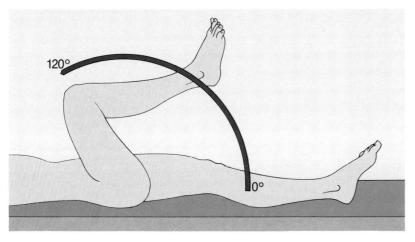

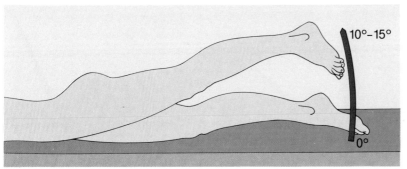

Figure 4.1 Flexion-extension of the hip. In the supine position, the hip can be flexed to 80°–90° with the knee extended (*top*) and to 120° with the knee flexed (*center*). With the patient prone, the hip can be extended 10°–15° (*bottom*). Extension is one of the first motions to be lost in arthritis of the hip, and will result in the development of a limp.

abduction-adduction (Fig. 4.2), and internal-external rotation (Fig. 4.3). In patients with osteoarthritis of the hip, the first motion lost is extension, followed by external rotation and abduction. Loss of motion occurs regardless of the underlying pathology.

A simple test for detecting disease in the hip joint without differentiating the extent of limitation in a specific motion is the heel-to-knee test (Patrick's maneuver or fabere sign) (Fig. 4.4). The motions utilized in this test are flexion, abduction, external rotation, and at the completion of the test, extension. (The initial letters of these motions were combined by Patrick to yield the acronym, *fabere.*) The hip

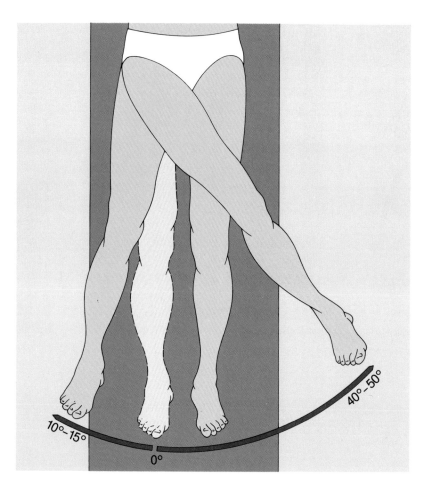

Figure 4.2 Abduction-adduction of the hip. With the patient supine, abduction of the hip should be between 40° and 50°; adduction should be between 10° and 15°. Foot should be in neutral position.

and the knee on the side to be tested are flexed so that the heel lies beside or on top of the opposite extended knee. The hip being examined is then abducted and externally rotated as far as possible. Any pain, muscle spasm, or limitation of motion in the region of the hip on the side being examined constitutes a positive result and suggests an abnormality in the hip. The test is negative when motion is normal and no pain or discomfort occurs.

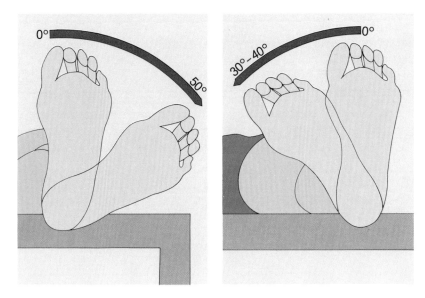

Figure 4.3 Internal-external rotation. With the patient in a supine position and the knee extended, rotation of the hip may be assessed by rotating the foot 50° laterally (*left*) and 30°–40° medially (*right*). Rotation is less sensitive to disease than is extension, but loss of rotation is also an early sign of arthritis of the hip.

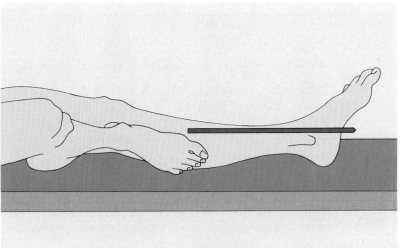

Figure 4.4 In Patrick's maneuver, the knee is flexed so that the heel of one leg approximates the knee of the other leg. Then, the leg is abducted, externally rotated, and extended so that the heel moves distally along the tibia.

A shortened extremity can also produce osteo-arthritis in the hip, so measurement of the patient's legs should be included in the physical examination. Measurement of leg length is performed most easily with the patient lying supine on a firm, level surface (Fig. 4.5). The length of each leg should be measured from the anterior-superior iliac spine to the prominence of the ipsilateral medial malleolus. The measuring tape crosses the anterior surface of the patella at its midline. Comparison of the measurements of the two legs usually reveals small differences in their length, but a difference of less than 1 cm does not affect the gait. A pelvic tilt may produce apparent but not actual shortening of the leg.

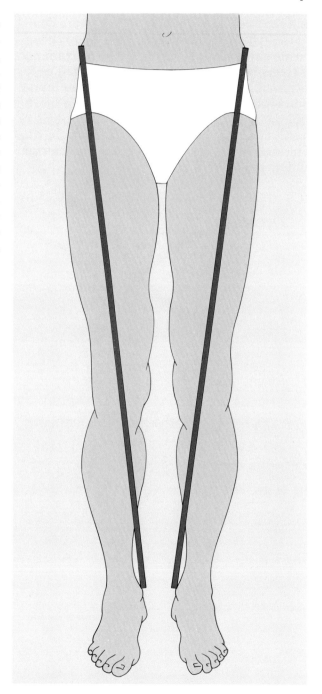

Figure 4.5 Leg length may be estimated by measuring from the anterior superior iliac spine to the prominence of the ipsilateral medial malleolus.

RADIOLOGIC FINDINGS

Unlike osteoarthritis in other joints, the radiologic findings in the hip correlate well with symptoms. When patients with osteoarthritis of the hip have radiographs taken of both hips, 78 percent show bilateral evidence of the disease.

When radiographs are classified by location of joint space narrowing or loss of cartilage, the predominant sites of osteoarthritis are found to be the superolateral, lateral, and superior aspects of the hip (Fig. 4.6). Early osteoarthritis can be seen to affect the superior compartment of the femoral acetabular articulation (Fig. 4.7), while in more advanced stages of the disease there may be extensive, nonuniform loss of joint space.

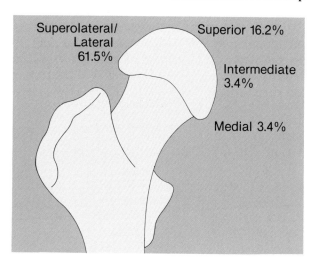

Figure 4.6   The predominant sites of joint space narrowing and cartilage loss in osteoarthritis of the hip. (Modified from Macys, Bullough, and Wilson, 1980)

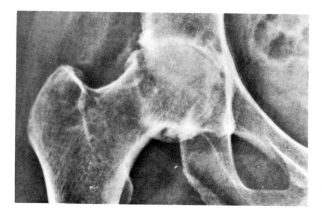

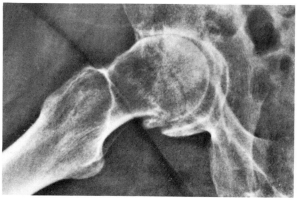

Figure 4.7   Anteroposterior radiograph of the hip (*left*) shows the typical signs of early osteoarthritis: joint space narrowing of the superior compartment, subchondral sclerosis, and minimal osteophyte formation. However, when a radiograph is taken of the hip in external rotation (*right*), the nonuniform joint space narrowing in the superior compartment becomes more obvious, and the medial compartment of the femoral acetabular articulation appears normal. This view will often demonstrate the earlier, more subtle changes associated with osteoarthritis before they are apparent on AP view.

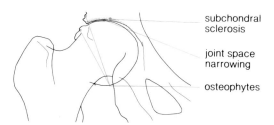

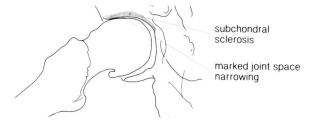

Osteophytes at the hip joint are a common occurrence, but of no prognostic value (Fig. 4.8).
In addition, buttressing of the neck of the
femur and remodeling of the head of the femur
may occur (Fig. 4.9).

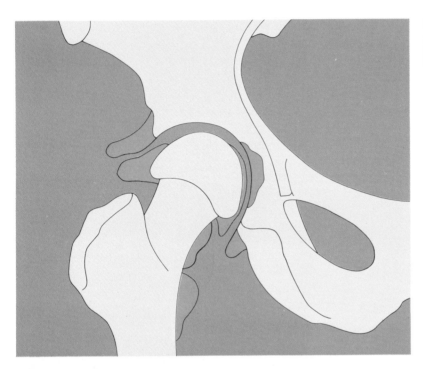

Figure 4.8 Distribution of osteo-
phytes in osteoarthritis of the hip.
(Modified from Macys, Bullough, and
Wilson, 1980)

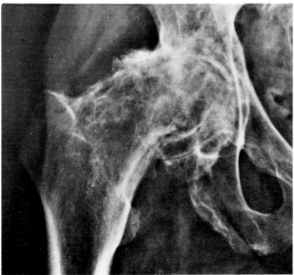

Figure 4.9 Radiograph of advanced osteoarthritis of the
hip shows large osteophytes buttressing the femoral neck,
gross deformity of the head of the femur, and essentially
complete loss of the joint space.

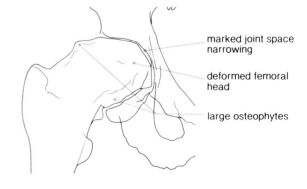

marked joint space
narrowing

deformed femoral
head

large osteophytes

Occasionally, large subchondral cysts may also be observed (Fig. 4.10). These cysts originate in the acetabulum, where they are frequently referred to as Egger's cysts. Since the cysts only appear after denudation of the overlying articular cartilage, this tends to support morphologic studies that suggest that osteoarthritis of the hip begins in the roof of the acetabulum rather than in the femoral head itself.

The medial compartment of the joint may rarely be involved (Fig. 4.11). When this is the case, disease is often bilateral.

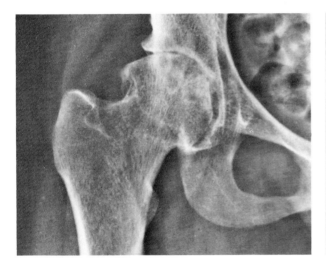

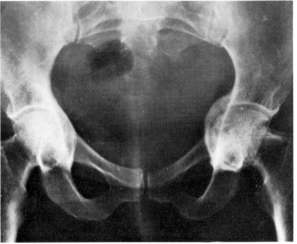

Figure 4.10   Radiograph of the hip shows large subchondral cysts involving the superior aspect of the joint.

Figure 4.11   In this radiograph, the medial hip compartments are involved, and there is resultant protrusion of the femoral head through the acetabulum. Marked sclerosis and thickening of the medial acetabular rim can be noted, especially on the right side. There is also increased bone thickening of the protruded portion of the acetabulum.

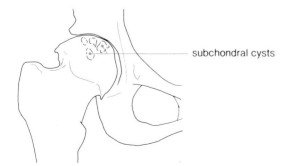

subchondral cysts

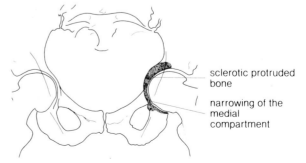

sclerotic protruded bone

narrowing of the medial compartment

In some cases there may be a marked inward bulging of the acetabulum, a condition known as protrusio acetabuli (Fig. 4.12). This may be found in association with Paget's disease, osteomalacia, and rheumatoid arthritis.

SECONDARY OSTEOARTHRITIS
Secondary osteoarthritis occurs most commonly in the hip, and in approximately 60 percent of patients the condition has resulted from a congenital or developmental abnormality including:

Hip dysplasias
Shallow acetabulum
Slipped capital femoral epiphysis
Legg-Calvé-Perthes disease
Femoral neck abnormalities
Primary protrusio acetabuli

Presentation of secondary osteoarthritis is usually 10 years earlier than the usual presentation of primary osteoarthritis, with the latter presenting in the middle of the seventh decade. The interval from onset to surgical intervention is longer in the primary form of the disease: 14 years prior to surgery as compared to 6 years in patients with secondary osteoarthritis.

Congenital dislocation of the hip with inadequate development of the acetabulum results in a shallow cavity on the lateral surface of the

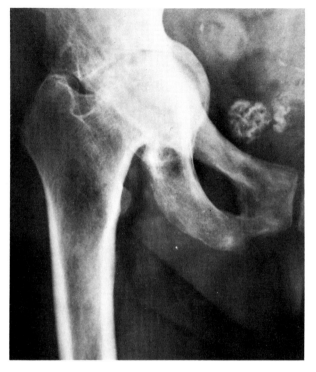

Figure 4.12   Anteroposterior radiograph of the hip demonstrates protrusion of the femoral head through the acetabulum, with marked sclerosis and thickening of the medial and superior acetabular rim. Coarsening of the trabeculae of the pelvic bone typical of Paget's disease can also be observed.

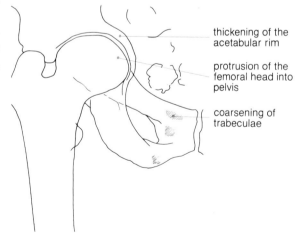

thickening of the acetabular rim

protrusion of the femoral head into pelvis

coarsening of trabeculae

os coxae. This cavity is directed laterally and anteriorly; consequently, the femoral head is insufficiently covered. Depending upon the degree of acetabular dysplasia, the femoral head may articulate with the superior aspect of the acetabulum, or a new "pseudoacetabulum" may be formed along the superior lateral aspect of the innominate bone (Fig. 4.13). Subluxation of the femoral head in children may result in the development of a limp, but symptoms may not appear until the teens. In less severe dislocations, the condition may first manifest as osteoarthritis of the hip in the fourth, fifth, or sixth decades.

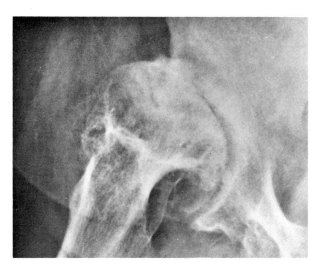
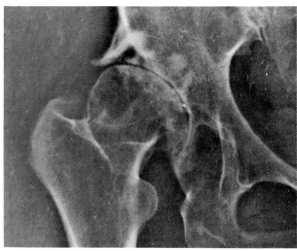

Figure 4.13 In acetabular dysplasia (*left*), the femoral head may articulate with the superior aspect of the acetabulum. In advanced dysplasia (*right*), the femoral head may slip so that there is a new "pseudoacetabulum" along the superior lateral aspect of the innominate bone.

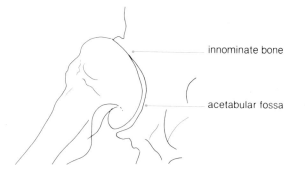
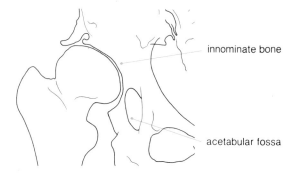

Slipped capital femoral epiphysis occurs in young adolescents, and may present as pain in the groin, buttock, thigh, or knee, sometimes resulting in a limping gait. Forceful internal rotation of the leg usually accentuates the pain. Patients may be asymptomatic for variable periods of time, and may not experience any pain until the fifth or sixth decades when osteoarthritis develops. Posterior slippage of the epiphysis can be noted in a lateral radiograph of the hip (Fig. 4.14). The resultant persistent deformity leads to secondary osteoarthritis.

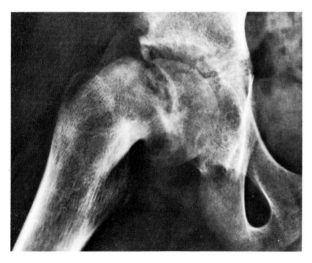
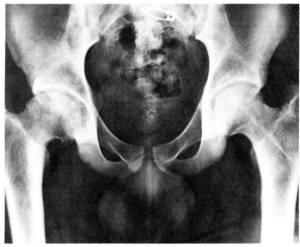

Figure 4.14 Frog-lateral view of the hip in a patient with slipped capital femoral epiphysis (*left*) reveals marked posterior displacement of the secondary center of ossification on the neck of the femur. An anteroposterior radiograph of this same hip, taken 13 years later (*right*), shows persis-

tent deformity of the femoral head, with a characteristic pistol-grip deformity (flattening of the head and shortening of the neck) and bony irregularity on the joint margin inferiorly. On the left hip one can note evidence of slight slippage and the residual tract of a nail used to fix the femoral head.

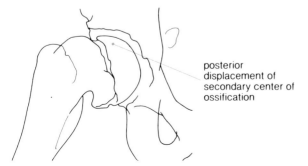
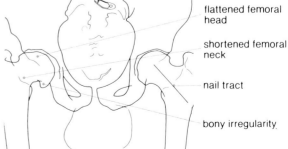

posterior displacement of secondary center of ossification

flattened femoral head

shortened femoral neck

nail tract

bony irregularity

Legg-Calvé-Perthes disease is an avascular necrosis of the proximal capital femoral epiphysis that occurs in children (Fig. 4.15). Peak incidence occurs between ages 4 and 8 years, mainly in boys. Distortion of the softened femoral head leads to gait abnormalities. In the third and fourth decades, persistent deformity of the femoral head leads to precocious osteoarthritis of the hip, the expected result of any condition associated with avascular necrosis.

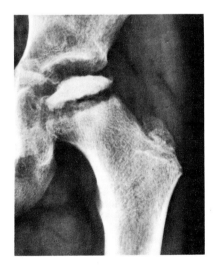 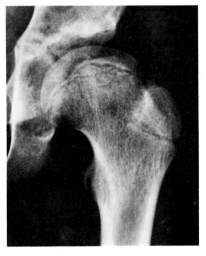 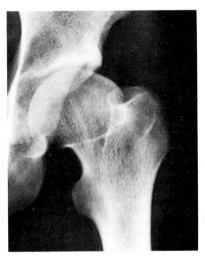

Figure 4.15 Radiograph of the left hip in a patient with Legg-Calvé-Perthes disease (*left*) shows widening of the joint space and growth plate, and increased density and collapse of the secondary center of ossification. Five years later (*center*), the secondary center of ossification has reformed and remodeled, but the hip appears relatively flattened and mushroom-shaped. One may also note some irregularity of the subchondral bone in the acetabular compartments. Ten years later (*right*), the radiograph shows flattening and deformity of the femoral head. The epiphyses are now fused, and there is a residual mushroom deformity of the femoral head with shortening of the femoral neck. The superior acetabular compartment also appears flattened.

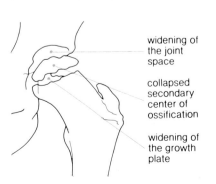 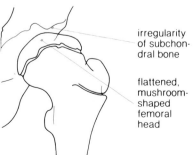 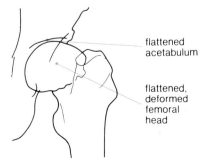

widening of the joint space

collapsed secondary center of ossification

widening of the growth plate

irregularity of subchondral bone

flattened, mushroom-shaped femoral head

flattened acetabulum

flattened, deformed femoral head

All patients with hemoglobinopathies (e.g., sickle cell anemia), systemic lupus erythematosus, or iatrogenic hypercortisonism may develop osteoarthritis of the hip secondary to osteonecrosis (Fig. 4.16).

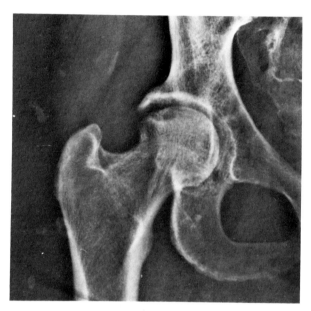 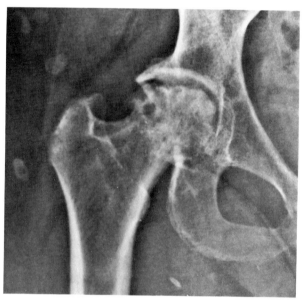

Figure 4.16   Radiograph of the hip (*left*) shows early signs of osteonecrosis. A well-defined subchondral zone of lucency is present, bound by an area of increased bone density. A localized cortical fracture is seen in the lucent zone. A large osteophyte can also be seen along the superior aspect of the femoral head. Radiograph of the same patient 6 years later (*right*) shows further progression of the osteonecrosis. Flattening and irregularity of the femoral head is now evident. In addition, there are extensive cystic and sclerotic changes of the femoral head.

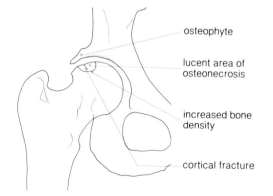 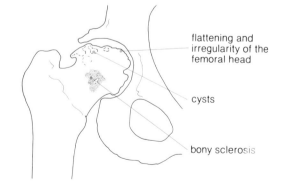

TREATMENT

Whether primary or secondary, the basis for treatment of patients with osteoarthritis of the hip remains the same: rest, rehabilitation, and analgesic drugs. (For a more detailed discussion of treatment, see Chapter 10.)

In advanced cases, prosthetic replacement of the osteoarthritic hip may be warranted. Total hip prostheses have been used for over 20 years in patients with severe degeneration and intractable pain (Fig. 4.17).

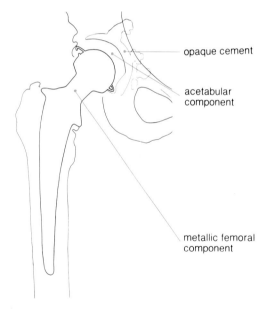

Figure 4.17 Radiograph showing a total hip prosthesis. The acetabular component is composed of ultra-high-density polyethylene plastic, and the femoral component is usually a metal alloy. The thickness of the acetabular component is that area that appears between the metallic femoral component and the opaque cement area.

opaque cement

acetabular component

metallic femoral component

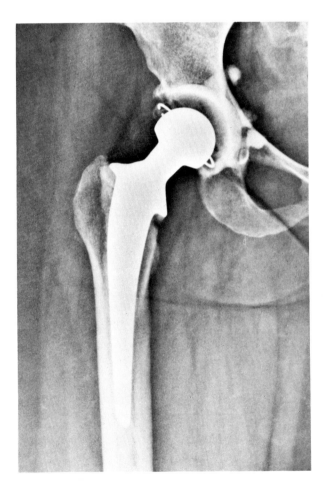

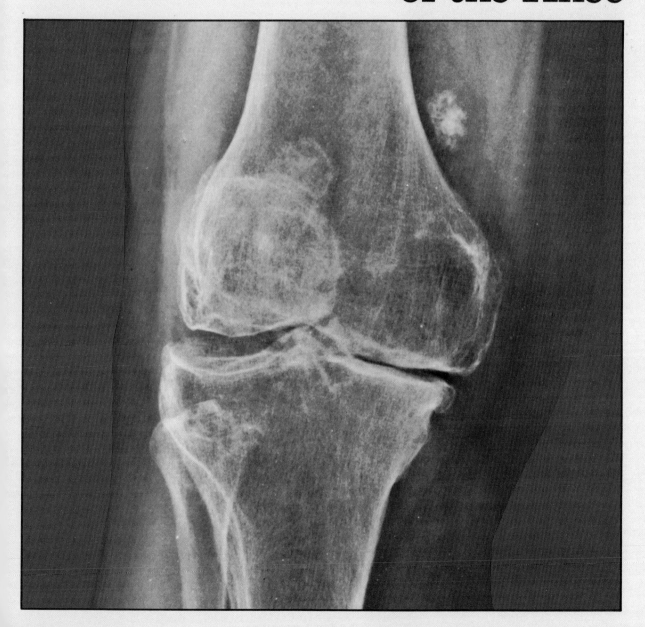

Osteoarthritis commonly occurs in the knee, and one or both knees may be the sole focus of the disease. Symptoms consist primarily of pain on motion which may be relieved by rest. Patients with osteoarthritis of the knee may also have difficulty kneeling or climbing stairs. Although symptoms do not usually occur in individuals under the age of 40, many of the causes of knee pain prior to that age may be risk factors for the later development of osteoarthritis (secondary osteoarthritis). Table 5.1 lists the differential diagnosis of knee pain, based on the age of the patient. Each of these disorders, with the exception of Osgood-Schlatter disease, may predispose the individual to osteoarthritis.

Osgood-Schlatter disease is a fragmentation of the tibial tubercle, and it usually presents as the insidious onset of knee pain in adolescent boys. Swelling of the tubercle or of the patellar tendon at the point at which it attaches to the tubercle can be noted. Although this is clearly a clinical diagnosis, a lateral radiograph may show soft-tissue changes overlying the tibial tubercle, and osseous irregularity of the tubercle within the tendinous insertion (Fig. 5.1). Treatment consists of avoidance of excessive physical activity, with resolution of the condition usually occurring in 6 to 8 weeks.

Table 5.1 Differential Diagnosis of Knee Pain (by Age)

18 Years or less

Osgood-Schlatter disease
Osteochondritis dissecans
Discoid lateral meniscus
Chondromalacia patellae

18–40

Trauma
    Ligamentous or meniscal damage
    Fracture
    Patellar dislocation
Rheumatoid arthritis
Other inflammatory arthropathies

40–80

Osteoarthritis
Osteonecrosis (aseptic necrosis)
Degenerative meniscal tears
Rheumatoid arthritis
Other inflammatory arthropathies

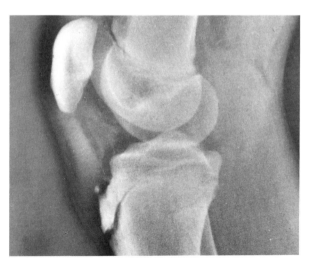

Figure 5.1 Lateral radiograph of the knee in an adolescent boy shows soft-tissue swelling over the tibial tubercle. One can also see displacement of an ossicle of bone anterior to the tubercle (Osgood-Schlatter disease).

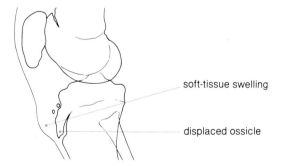

soft-tissue swelling

displaced ossicle

CONDITIONS PREDISPOSING TO OSTEOARTHRITIS OF THE KNEE

It is becoming increasingly evident that many cases of osteoarthritis in the knee begin with trauma to the ligaments or to the articular surfaces years before symptoms occur. These traumatic insults initiate a process of degeneration within any or all of the three compartments of the knee: the medial, patellofemoral, or lateral compartment.

Osteochondritis dissecans is a disorder of subchondral bone also commonly found in the knees of adolescents. A devitalized fragment of bone with its articular cartilage still present migrates from its original site, and it may separate partially or completely from the joint surfaces. If completely separated, the resultant loose body may lead to the locking of the joint. Osteochondritis is localized in the medial femoral condyle in 86 percent of cases (Fig. 5.2).

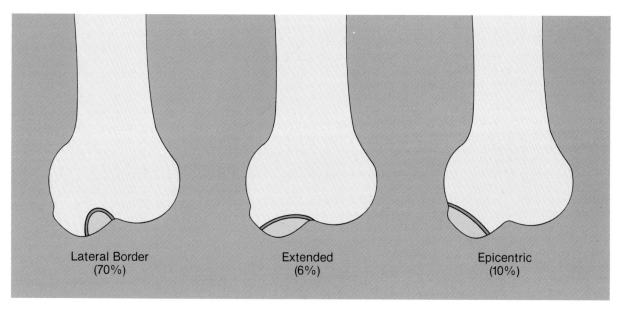

Lateral Border
(70%)

Extended
(6%)

Epicentric
(10%)

Figure 5.2 Osteochondritis dissecans usually occurs on the medial femoral condyle (86%). The classic site is on the lateral border of the medial condyle (70%), but it may occur at other sites as well.

A fragment of bone with a sharply demarcated border can be observed radiographically (Fig. 5.3).

Articular cartilage damage in the patellofemoral joint is considered part of the normal aging process. However, when it occurs prematurely, it is termed *chondromalacia patellae*, a morbid softening, fissuring, and degeneration of the articular surface of the patella. Chondromalacia is usually secondary to a mechanical disturbance, either patellar subluxation or mild patellar malalignment, and usually occurs in young girls.

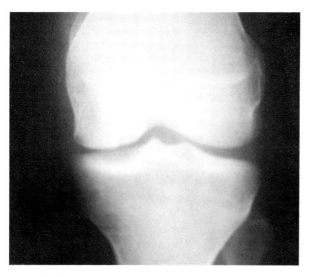
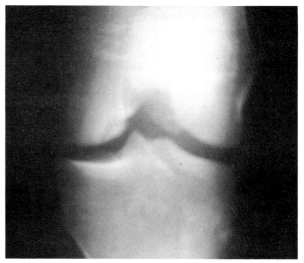

Figure 5.3   Anteroposterior radiograph of the knee (*left*) demonstrates classic osteochondritis dissecans, with a curvilinear lucency along the lateral border of the medial femoral condyle. A tunnel view (*right*) obtained with the knee in 90° of flexion shows more clearly the area of osteochondritis dissecans. A zone of sclerotic reactive bone can be seen bordering the necrotic fragment.

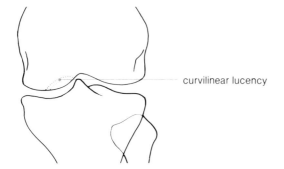
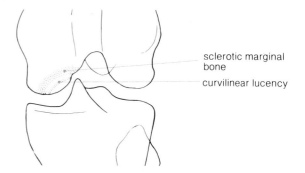

curvilinear lucency

sclerotic marginal bone

curvilinear lucency

Pain and crepitation occur from pressure against the patella or downward resistance upon the patella during a forceful quadriceps contraction. In early chondromalacia patellae, there may be only minimal irregularity of the posterior surface of the patella (Fig. 5.4). In advanced cases, lateral radiographs may show a markedly irregular posterior surface and/or marginal osteophytes (Fig. 5.5). Exercise has been found to relieve symptoms in a considerable number of patients. For those not helped by the exercises, realignment of the patella may be indicated.

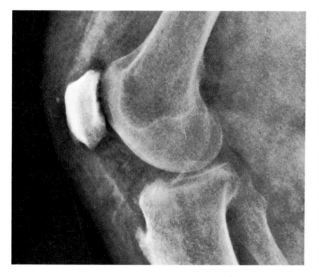

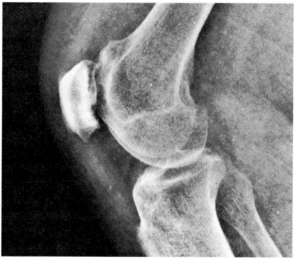

Figure 5.4   Lateral radiograph of the knee in early chondromalacia patellae shows minimal irregularity of the posterior surface of the patella. The joint space appears to be entirely normal.

Figure 5.5   Lateral radiograph of the knee shows advanced chondromalacia patellae, with narrowing of the joint space, irregularity, marginal osteophytes, and subchondral bony sclerosis.

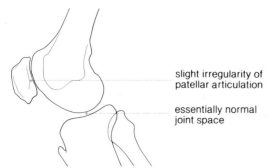

slight irregularity of patellar articulation

essentially normal joint space

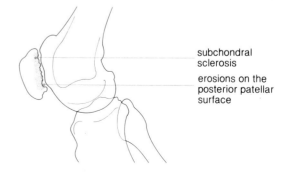

subchondral sclerosis

erosions on the posterior patellar surface

Trauma may ultimately lead to osteoarthritis as a result of the loss of stability and integrity in the joint. The stability and integrity of the knee joint depend primarily upon the integrity of the surrounding muscles and ligaments, i.e., the cruciates, the collaterals, and the joint capsule. The medial collateral ligament is superficial, and extends from the medial femoral epicondyle to the tibia. The lateral collateral

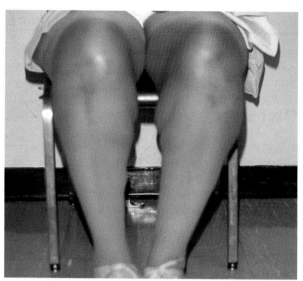

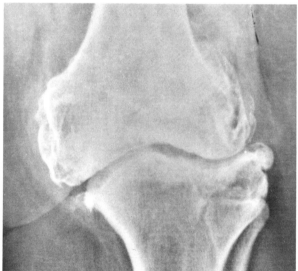

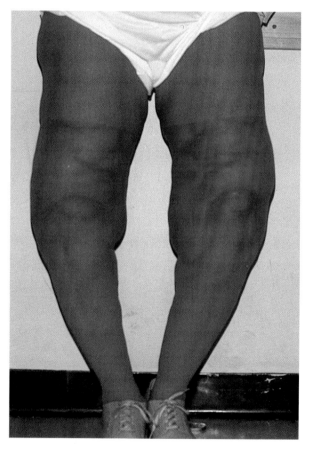

Figure 5.6 The obese patient above has a marked genu varus deformity of both knees, which is readily apparent in standing photographs. The deformity is less apparent in sitting photographs (*top right*). An anteroposterior radiograph of this patient's knee (*bottom right*) shows marked medial and lateral compartment degenerative changes, with narrowing of the medial compartment, extensive osteophyte formation, and subchondral bony sclerosis.

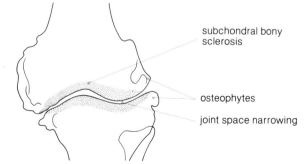

subchondral bony sclerosis

osteophytes

joint space narrowing

ligament extends from the lateral femoral epicondyle to the head of the fibula. With normal articular cartilage and collateral ligaments, there should be less than 5° of lateral movement in the extended knee. Increased lateral motion may signal either ligamentous laxity or degeneration of the cartilage. Disproportionate degenerative changes localized to the medial or lateral aspects of the knee may lead to secondary genu varum (bowlegs) or genu valgum (knock-knees) with joint instability and subluxation.

Instability is further aggravated by laxity of the collateral ligaments. It is important to compare the degree of varus or valgus deformity during weight bearing and at rest. If a change in varus alignment or an increase in the degree of deformity occurs during weight bearing, it is evidence of cartilage loss and compartment deformity rather than ligamentous laxity (Fig. 5.6).

In patients with Morquio's syndrome, a mucopolysaccharide storage disease, congenital ligamentous laxity at the knee joint leads to an early and severe genu valgus deformity and, ultimately, to secondary osteoarthritis of the knee (Fig. 5.7).

Osteonecrosis refers to a focal segment of bone death which is usually subchondral in origin. The clinical disabilities that result from osteonecrosis are not directly related to bone tissue pathology, but rather to structural changes that develop in the articular surface. The sudden onset of pain in the knee and a rather rapid progressive syndrome of osteoarthritis may occur in middle-aged women with osteonecrosis of the femoral condyle.

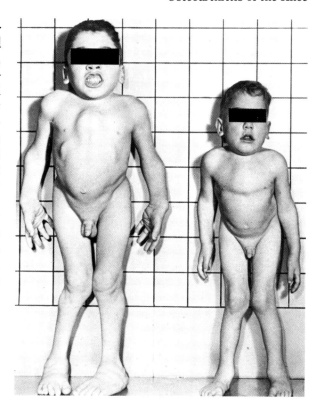

Figure 5.7 These patients with Morquio's syndrome have marked genu valgum secondary to ligamentous laxity, which ultimately leads to degenerative changes in the knees. (Courtesy of Dr. David Kaplan)

Osteonecrosis may be differentiated on the basis of a technetium scan which demonstrates localized increased uptake in the osteonecrotic area on the femoral condyle, but not on the tibial aspect of the joint (Fig. 5.8). In osteoarthritis, the same degree of increased uptake would be seen on both the femoral and tibial aspects of the joint. Eventually, osteonecrosis leads to osteoarthritis and the destruction of the joint (Fig. 5.9). The causes of osteonecrosis in the knee are the same as those that cause the disease in the hip and elsewhere (Table 5.2).

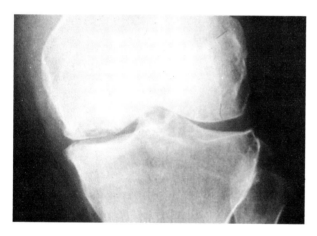

Figure 5.8   Radiograph (*left*) of the knee in a 64-year-old female with osteonecrosis reveals a subchondral focus of lysis in the medial femoral condyle. A technetium bone scan (*right*) demonstrates a focal area of high uptake over the medial femoral condyle which corresponds to the area of lysis seen in the radiograph. Note that the tibial aspect of the medial compartment does not show increased uptake.

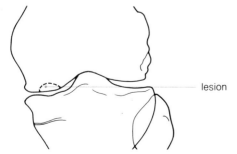

lesion

CLINICAL SIGNS AND FEATURES

The knee joint is supported by both ligaments and fibrocartilaginous menisci, each of which is important in evaluating the integrity of the joint. The paired cruciate ligaments are named according to their tibial attachments. The anterior cruciate ligament extends from its anterior medial tibial attachment to the lateral femoral condyle. It prevents abnormal exter-

Table 5.2   Causes of Osteonecrosis

Trauma
Excess glucocorticosteroids
   Steroid therapy
   Cushing's syndrome
Systemic lupus erythematosus
Hemoglobinopathies
   S-S, S-C, others
Metabolic disorders
   Gout and hyperuricemia
   Gaucher's disease
   Alcoholism
   Caisson disease
   Fat embolism
Idiopathic causes (no known association)

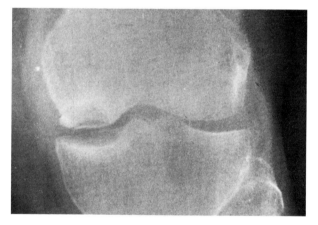
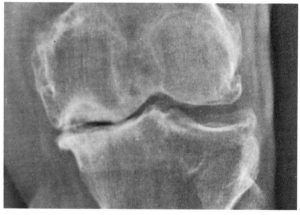

Figure 5.9   In early osteonecrosis (*left*), an anteroposterior radiograph shows a radiolucent subcortical crescent. The joint space remains essentially normal. In advanced osteonecrosis (*right*), a crescentic lucency with a surrounding zone of increased radiodensity is clearly evident. In addition, there are marked secondary degenerative changes, with joint space narrowing of the affected (medial) compartment and osteophyte formation at the joint margin and on the tibial plateau.

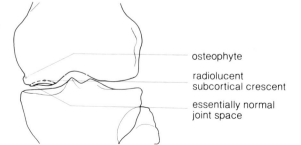

osteophyte
radiolucent subcortical crescent
essentially normal joint space

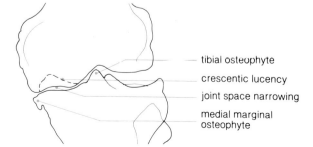

tibial osteophyte
crescentic lucency
joint space narrowing
medial marginal osteophyte

nal rotation, stabilizes the knee in extension, and prevents hyperextension (Fig. 5.10). The posterior cruciate ligament extends from the posterior aspect of the tibia to the medial femoral condyle. It prevents excessive internal rotation and aids normal knee flexion (Fig. 5.11). Instability in the hyperextended knee indicates damage to the cruciates.

The drawer test for cruciate instability is performed with the patient's knee flexed to 90° and the foot also flexed (Fig. 5.12). When a tear has occurred in the anterior cruciate ligament, the tibia moves forward.

The menisci are curved, wedge-shaped, fibrocartilaginous structures that assist in distributing pressure between the femur and the tibia. They also increase the elasticity of the joint and assist in its lubrication. The medial meniscus is larger and more susceptible to injury than the lateral meniscus.

The importance of the meniscus in the pathogenesis of osteoarthritis of the knee was recognized as early as 1942, when Bennett, Waine, and Bauer reported their observations at autopsy of degenerative changes in 63 knee joints at various ages. They noted that "in every subject beyond the age of fifteen some degeneration of the knee joint was observable," and that "the earliest detectable lesions

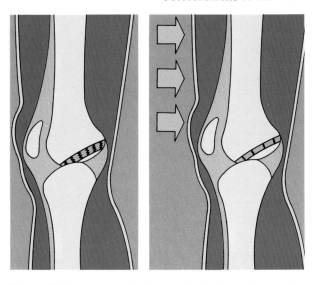

Figure 5.10   Schematic diagram (*left*) shows the anterior cruciate ligament attached anteriorly to the intercondyloid eminence of the tibia and extending posteriorly to the lateral femoral condyle. When force (*arrows*) is applied to the femur (*right*), the anterior cruciate ligament prevents the tibia from moving forward on the femur and thus prevents hyperextension of the knee.

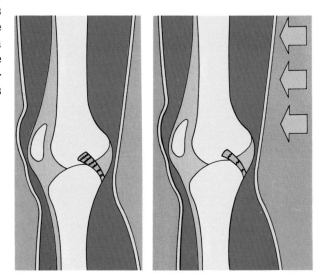

Figure 5.11   Schematic diagram (*left*) shows the posterior cruciate ligament attached to the posterior intercondyloid fossa of the tibia and to the lateral meniscus. It then passes anteriorly to the medial femoral condyle. When a pulling force (*arrows*) is applied at the femur (*right*), the posterior cruciate ligament keeps the tibia from moving backward on the femur.

are located in areas bearing the brunt of physiological use, that is, the patella and the exposed weight bearing portions of the femoral and tibial condyles." The tibial condyles "showed somewhat greater abnormalities than were seen in other portions of the joints . . . and these changes were confined entirely to the weight bearing parts not covered by the menisci." In fact, areas of cartilage which are consistently in contact and which are loaded during most activities are well-preserved. The loss of the meniscus following surgical removal results in abnormal patterns of loading and, ultimately, in progressive osteoarthritis.

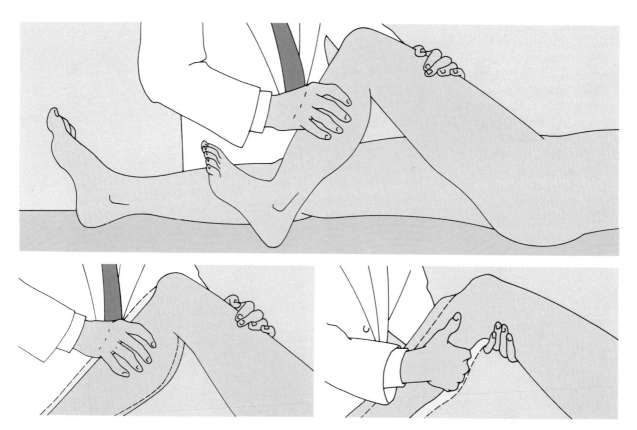

Figure 5.12   The drawer test for cruciate ligaments. With the patient supine, the knee flexed, and the foot flexed on the examining table, the examiner attempts to move the lower leg in a horizontal direction toward the hip. Under normal conditions, there would be little or no movement of the tibia upon the femur. With a tear of the posterior cruciate, the tibia will move back toward the femur (*left*). With a tear of the anterior cruciate, the tibia will move anteriorly when the force of the examiner's hand is pulling the tibia away from the body (*right*).

The pain of meniscus injury is usually severe and sudden, with swelling (effusion) occurring within hours of the injury. Locking of the joint is rare on initial injury, as the tear is usually in the posterior third of the meniscus, with no displacement or bending of the cartilage. However, where there are severe initial tears or repeated tearing injuries, locking of the knee can result, thereby preventing its full extension. Only half the patients with meniscal injuries describe a history of locking. Progressive articular damage is inevitable following meniscal tears.

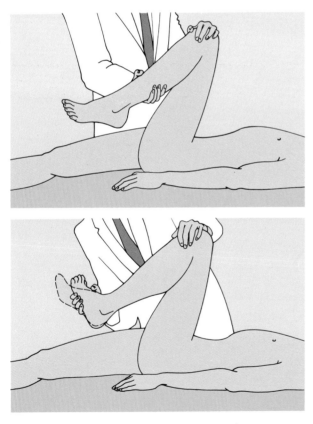

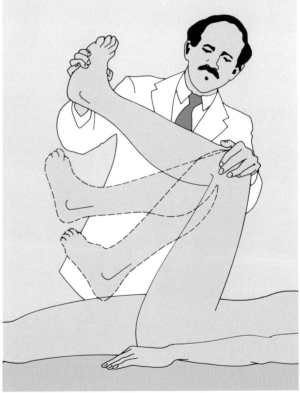

Figure 5.13   The McMurray sign. (*Left*) With the patient in the supine position, the knee is fully flexed so that the heel touches the buttocks. To test the lateral meniscus, the leg is internally rotated, and the knee is extended—with rotation forcefully maintained. Then the knee is extended to 90° of flexion, and if there is a meniscal tear, a painful click will oc-

Several signs of meniscal injury have been described, and they may assist in confirming the diagnosis. To examine for the McMurray sign (Fig. 5.13), place the patient in a recumbent position, with the knee flexed until the heel approaches the buttocks. The leg should be externally rotated upon the femur to test the medial meniscus. The leg is then gradually extended, with rotation forcefully maintained. The test is valid only during extension to 90° of flexion, and it does not diagnose tears in the anterior third of the meniscus. Pain and an audible click occur if the test is positive.

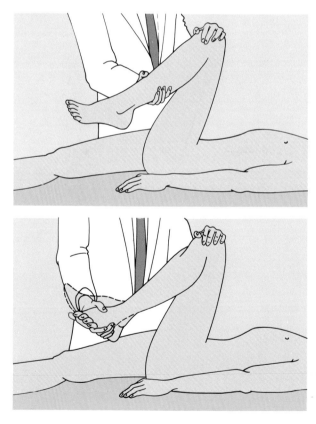

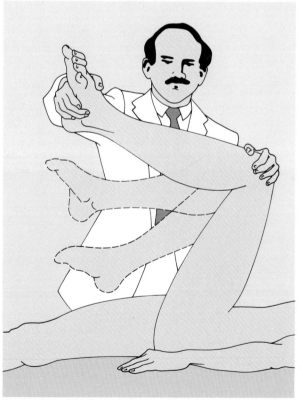

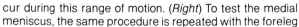

cur during this range of motion. (*Right*) To test the medial meniscus, the same procedure is repeated with the foreleg held in forced external rotation. The test does not diagnose tears in the anterior third of the meniscus.

The Apley test differentiates a meniscal lesion from a capsular or ligamentous injury (Fig. 5.14). With the patient prone, the knee is flexed at 90°, and the leg is rotated with simultaneous upward traction. If pain results from this maneuver, a capsular or ligamentous injury is likely. If rotation of the bent knee with downward pressure causes pain or a clicking sound, a meniscal injury is indicated.

Steinmann's "tenderness displacement sign" signals a meniscal injury if tenderness is displaced posteriorly as the knee is flexed, and anteriorly as the knee is extended (Fig. 5.15). The site of tenderness does not shift in patients with osteoarthritis of the knee.

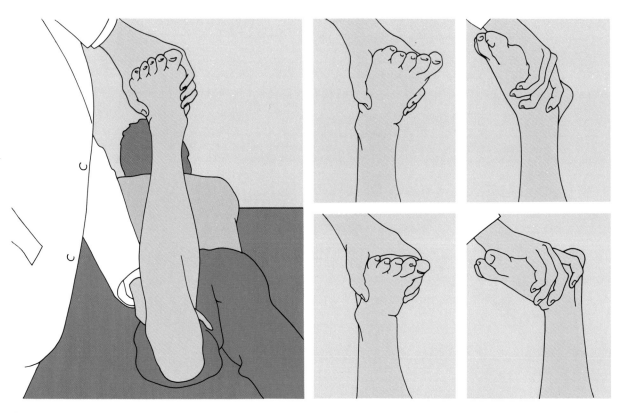

Figure 5.14   The Apley test. With the patient prone and the knee flexed to 90°, the leg is internally or externally rotated with simultaneous upward traction (*top*). Pain during the maneuver implies capsular or ligamentous injury. If rotation with downward pressure (*bottom*) causes pain or a click, a meniscal injury is indicated.

Physical findings in patients with osteoarthritis of the knee include local tenderness and a sense of grating or crackling (described as crepitus) that accompanies both active and passive meniscal movements. Crepitus presumably results from gross surface incongruities and eburnation of bone. Joint enlargements and deformity occur in both bone and soft tissue, with preservation of at least serviceable function. Synovial effusions are common, and the synovial fluid has normal viscosity and a normal cell count.

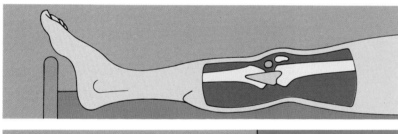

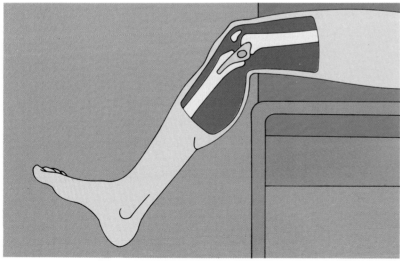

Figure 5.15 Steinmann's tenderness displacement sign. In patients with meniscal injuries, tenderness (represented by blue dot) occurs anteriorly when the knee is extended (*top*). As the knee is flexed, tenderness moves posteriorly toward the collateral ligament (*bottom*).

RADIOLOGIC FEATURES

Osteoarthritis of the knee is characterized radiologically by a nonuniform loss of cartilage, usually in the medial or patellofemoral compartment (or both). The formation of osteophytes, however, is most often generalized. Osteophytes commonly occur at the margins of the joints, and in areas of capsular recesses such as the middle of the tibial plateau (Fig. 5.16).

In patients with mild osteoarthritis, anteroposterior weight-bearing radiologic films should be obtained to assess the extent of cartilage loss. Radiographs taken with the patient in a reclining position may well show a normal joint space, but in standing radiographs the medial compartment may be entirely absent (Fig. 5.17).

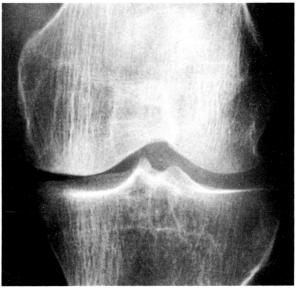

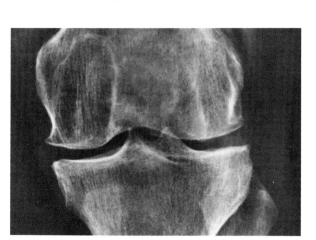

Figure 5.16 Radiograph shows osteophytes present along the margins of the articular surfaces, most predominantly along the medial aspect of the medial femorotibial compartment.

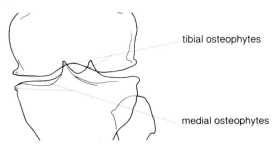

tibial osteophytes

medial osteophytes

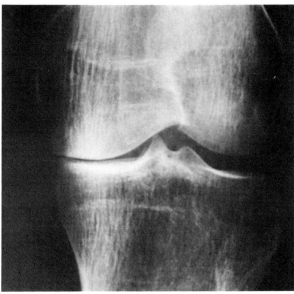

Figure 5.17 Radiograph of the knee in an elderly osteoarthritic patient, taken with the patient in a supine position (*top*), reveals an apparently normal joint space with some evidence of subchondral bony sclerosis in both the medial femoral condyle and the medial tibial plateau. However, a radiograph of the same knee with the patient standing (*bottom*) reveals severe joint space narrowing, a manifestation of osteoarthritis which only becomes apparent when the joint is subjected to load-bearing. (From Insall, 1984)

With a moderate degree of osteoarthritis, a loss of cartilage and evident narrowing of the joint space in the medial compartment can be noted on a standard reclining radiograph (Fig. 5.18). In advanced osteoarthritis, there also may be flattening and irregularity of the articular surfaces. The lateral compartment may be virtually normal.

Focal cartilage loss is frequently accompanied by discrete, local subchondral sclerosis (eburnation), again most commonly in the medial tibial plateau (Fig. 5.19). Significant narrowing of the joint space in the medial compartment can be clearly seen, and the subchondral bone displays increased density on the tibial aspect.

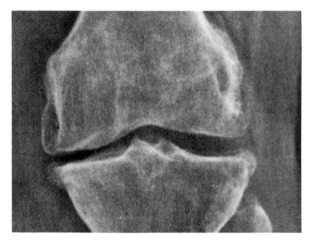

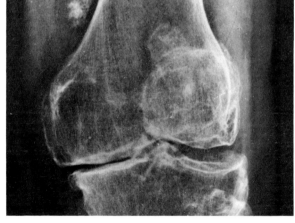

Figure 5.18 In this radiograph, osteophytes, joint space narrowing, and subchondral tibial sclerosis are evident in the medial compartment. Flattening of the articular surfaces, shown here, is often seen in advanced osteoarthritis.

Figure 5.19 Radiograph shows extensive subchondral sclerosis and marked narrowing of the medial compartment. Irregularity of all the articular surfaces is also seen.

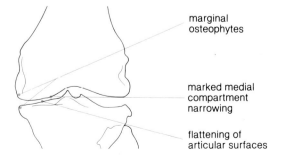

marginal osteophytes

marked medial compartment narrowing

flattening of articular surfaces

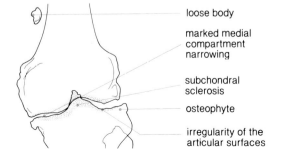

loose body

marked medial compartment narrowing

subchondral sclerosis

osteophyte

irregularity of the articular surfaces

After significant loss of cartilage, remodeling occurs and produces a beveled or scalloped appearance in the tibial plateau, with flattening of the femoral condyle. These advanced changes are frequently associated with some type of subluxation, such as widening of the joint, horizontal translocation, or angular deviation (Fig. 5.20).

Small pieces of cartilage may be dislodged into the synovial fluid and subsequently develop into "loose bodies" or "mice" (Figs. 5.19, 5.21, and 5.22). In Figures 5.21 and 5.22, one may note large loose bodies within the suprapatellar bursa. The loose bodies can result in locking of the joint and episodic severe knee pain; they may ultimately require surgical removal.

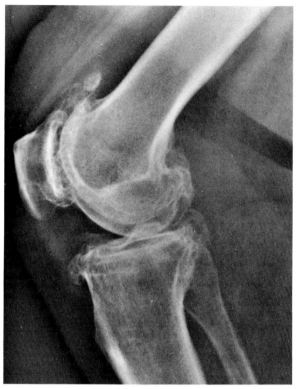

Figure 5.21   Lateral radiograph shows large osteophytes along the margins of all the articular surfaces. A large loose body is present in the suprapatellar bursa.

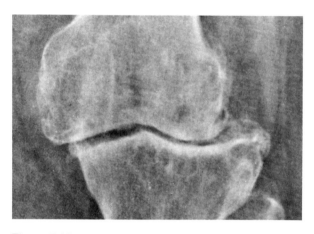

Figure 5.20   Radiograph shows advanced osteoarthritis, with subluxation and angulation of the femoral condyle on the tibia (genu varum). In addition, there is extensive joint space narrowing of both the medial and lateral compartments, extensive osteophyte formation, and subchondral sclerosis.

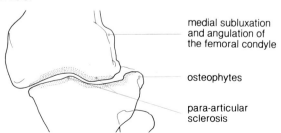

medial subluxation
and angulation of
the femoral condyle

osteophytes

para-articular
sclerosis

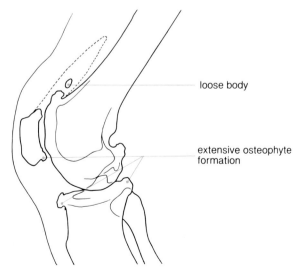

loose body

extensive osteophyte
formation

TREATMENT

Several forms of surgery may be beneficial in patients with advanced osteoarthritis of the knee. Joint debridement (including the removal of large osteophytes, torn menisci, and loose bodies) may relieve pain and retard the degenerative process. An osteotomy may serve to relieve pain and disability by redistributing weight and external stresses more optimally over the joint surfaces.

In advanced osteoarthritis, a total prosthetic replacement of the knee (Fig. 5.23) may provide a greater degree of motion and stability, as well as alleviate pain. These prostheses have become more sophisticated, and they are now approaching the level of success achieved in total hip replacement procedures.

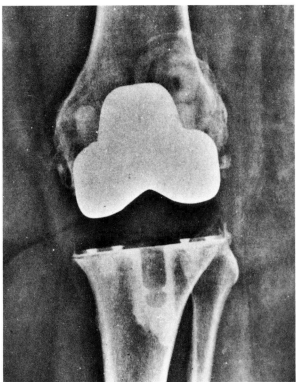

Figure 5.23   Radiograph shows total femoral and tibial joint replacement. The prosthesis shown here is commercially available, combining a metal alloy femoral condyle with a high-molecular-weight polyethylene tibial plateau.

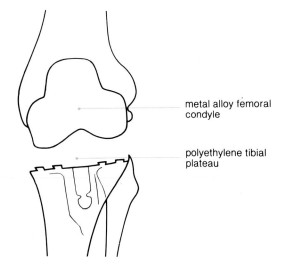

metal alloy femoral condyle

polyethylene tibial plateau

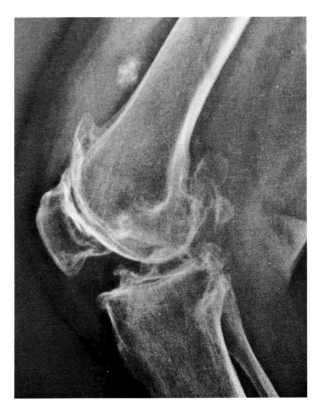

Figure 5.22   Lateral radiograph shows a large, distinctive ossified loose body in the suprapatellar bursa.

6
Osteoarthritis
of the Foot

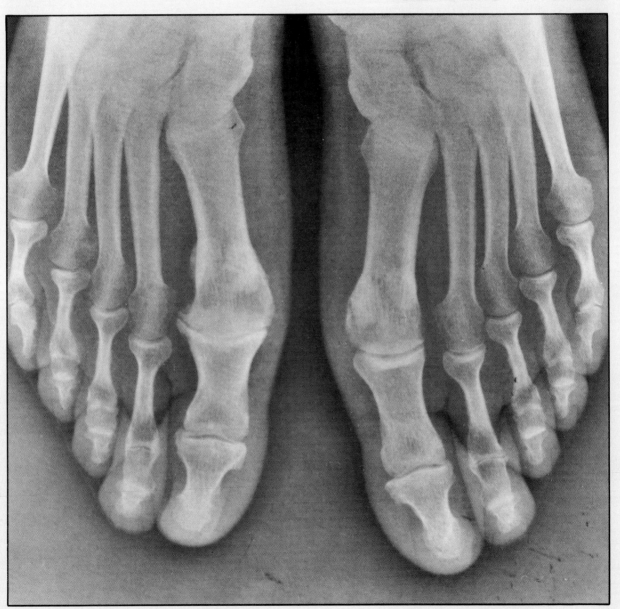

Painful conditions of the foot usually originate in the soft tissues (e.g., muscles, ligaments, and tendons) rather than in the joints. In most cases the inciting incident will be apparent, as will a local lesion.

Although osteoarthritis of the foot is most commonly found in the first metatarsophalangeal joint, it may also occur at other sites and be a secondary complication of ligamentous or sports-related injuries.

OSTEOARTHRITIS OF THE FIRST METATARSOPHALANGEAL JOINT

A patient with osteoarthritis of the first metatarsophalangeal (MTP) joint presents with pain in the toe, especially following prolonged walking or strenuous physical activity. Early physical findings may be absent, or they may be present in the form of small bony irregularities along the medial aspect of the first MTP joint, representing early osteophyte formation (Fig. 6.1). As the degenerative process progresses in more advanced osteoarthritis, there may be marked osteophyte formation and

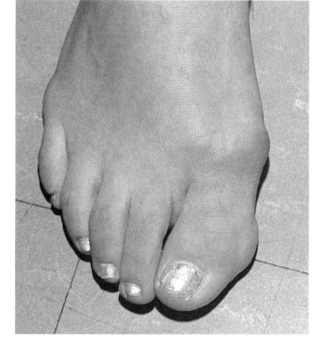

Figure 6.2   This photograph of a slightly more advanced stage of osteoarthritis reveals marked osteophyte formation as well as localized swelling and erythema (bunion) over the medial aspect of the first MTP joint.

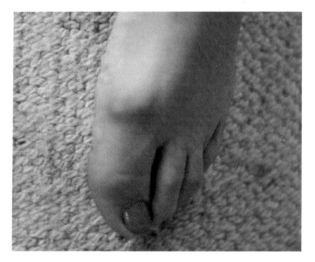

Figure 6.1   This photograph shows a foot in an early stage of osteoarthritis. Note the slight bony enlargement (osteophyte formation) along the medial aspect of the first MTP joint.

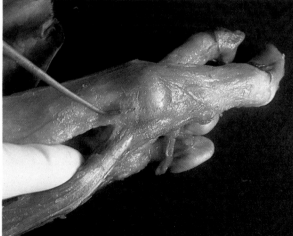

Figure 6.3   Gross dissection of the foot demonstrates a large bony osteophyte over the medial aspect of the first metatarsal bone.

local erythema over the first MTP joint (Fig. 6.2). Pathologically, large exuberant osteophytes can be noted on the medial aspect of the first metatarsal bone (Fig. 6.3).

On radiologic examination, a loss of joint space, para-articular sclerosis, and osteophyte formation are evident (Fig. 6.4).

Figure 6.4   Anteroposterior *(top)* and lateral *(bottom)* radiographs of the first phalanx show nonuniform loss of joint space, minimal para-articular sclerosis, and osteophyte formation, the latter being most obvious on lateral view.

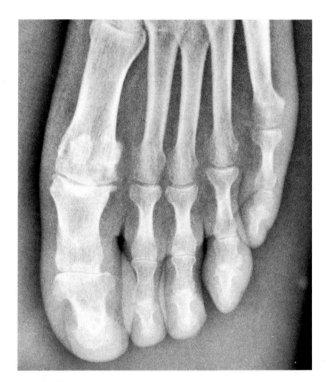

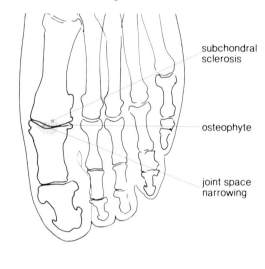

subchondral sclerosis

osteophyte

joint space narrowing

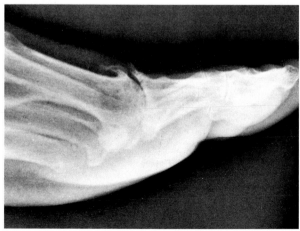

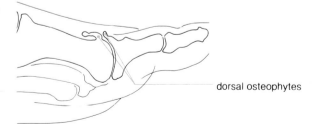

dorsal osteophytes

Histologically, extensive nonuniform joint space narrowing and subchondral sclerosis can be noted (Fig. 6.5). Large subchondral cysts may also develop (Fig. 6.6), and may occasionally be difficult to distinguish from the punched-out lesions of gout (Fig. 6.7). In such a case, the clinical picture should establish the diagnosis. Osteoarthritis is an insidious process with mild to moderate pain and characteristic deformity of the first MTP joint, whereas gout is an episodic disease characterized by intense, severe pain, marked erythema, and soft-tissue swelling (Fig. 6.8).

Congenital or developmental abnormalities of the first MTP joint, such as hallux valgus,

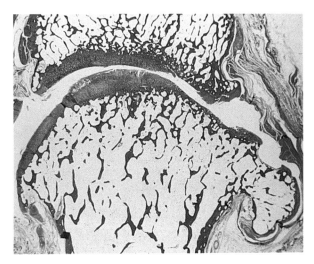

Figure 6.5 In this photomicrograph of the first MTP joint one may note severe, nonuniform joint space narrowing with areas of marked cartilage degeneration and osteophyte formation. The areas of intense staining beneath the cartilage represent subchondral sclerosis. (Courtesy of the Arthritis Foundation Teaching Collection)

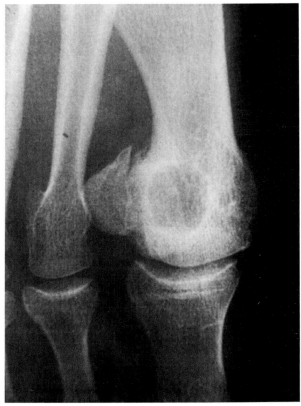

Figure 6.6 Radiograph shows a large subchondral cyst in the head of the first metatarsal bone. Such a cyst, commonly observed in osteoarthritis, usually has a discrete margin and does not communicate with the cortex.

may predispose to osteoarthritis of that joint. Conversely, osteoarthritis may well bring about the hallux valgus deformity by destroying the first MTP joint, thus creating the progressive lateral subluxation of the first digit.

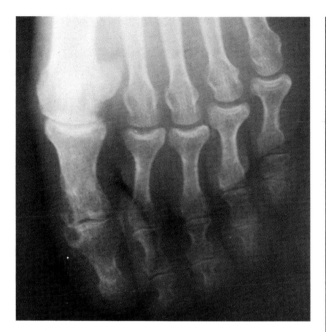

Figure 6.7 Radiograph shows a punched-out lesion at the interphalangeal joint of the first phalanx, characteristic of tophaceous gout. Note that the lesion communicates with the cortex and has a distinguishing overhanging ridge, in contrast to the subchondral cyst associated with osteoarthritis.

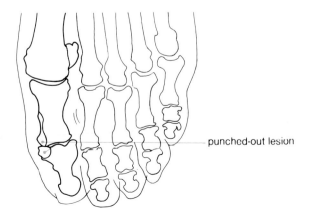

punched-out lesion

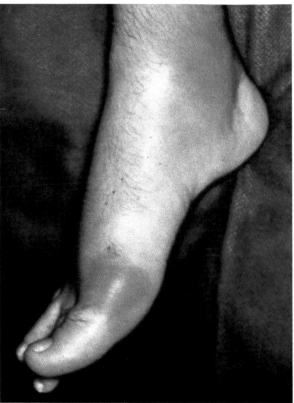

Figure 6.8 On clinical examination, gouty arthritis of the first MTP joint is usually quite intense, with severe pain at rest, marked erythema, and extensive soft-tissue swelling both locally and over the dorsum of the foot. (Courtesy of the Arthritis Foundation Teaching Collection)

Hallux valgus, a medial deviation of the first phalanx, is commonly associated with osteoarthritis of the first MTP joint. This deformity is characterized by three major clinicopathologic changes:

1. The large toe angulates toward the second toe (Fig. 6.9).
2. The medial portion of the first metatarsal head enlarges (Fig. 6.10).
3. The bursa over the medial aspect of the joint becomes inflamed and thick-walled (Fig. 6.11).

If hallux valgus occurs in a young person, predisposing genetic factors such as a varus deformity of the first metatarsal or a depressed metatarsal arch may be the underlying cause. Treatment should be aimed at retarding the degenerative process that occurs secondary to abnormal stresses at the first MTP joint. The patient should wear a wide shoe with a flat heel, and a stabilizing splint should be worn at night. In older patients in whom molded shoes and arch supports have been unsuccessful, surgical correction may be warranted.

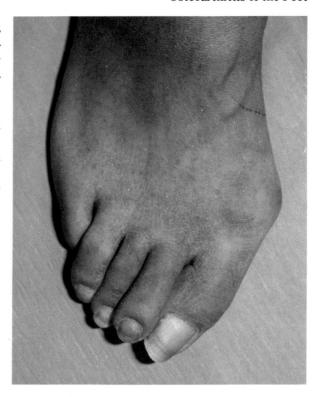

Figure 6.9 Hallux valgus deformity: As seen in this photograph, the first phalanx is markedly angulated toward the second toe, and may actually override the second toe in severe cases.

Figure 6.10 Hallux valgus deformity: Radiograph of the foot shows marked angulation of the first phalanx. Note the bony hypertrophy of the medial aspect of the head of the first metatarsal bone.

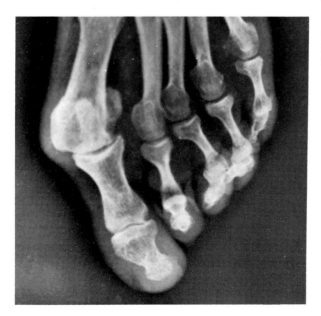

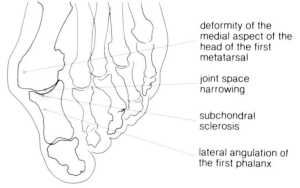

deformity of the medial aspect of the head of the first metatarsal

joint space narrowing

subchondral sclerosis

lateral angulation of the first phalanx

Alternately, there may be progressive loss of motion of the first MTP joint, resulting in hallux rigidus deformity. The patient cannot dorsiflex the toe, which interferes with smooth takeoff during ambulation. The partially rigid toe may be painful, but once the fusion is complete, the pain may disappear.

Several developmental abnormalities have been associated with the finding of hallux rigidus, specifically doral extension of the first metatarsal, an abnormally long first metatarsal, and pronation of the forefoot. These abnormalities in combination with trauma probably lead to osteochondritis dissecans on the superior aspect of the articular surface of the first metatarsal. However, this lesion may not be appreciated radiographically because the cleavage lesion occurs without the attachment of subchondral bone, and ultimately the radiographic findings are those of osteoarthritis.

Usually, patients with hallux rigidus complain of pain elsewhere in the foot, resulting from attempts to avoid stress on the big toe. The patient shifts weight to the outer border of the foot, and consequently "rolls off" the head of the fifth metatarsal during walking. Pressure symptoms occur under the fourth and fifth metatarsals as well as at the first metatarsal. Treatment consists of preventing stress on the rigid toe by placing a steel plate in the sole of the shoe to prevent bending, and a rocker bar on the bottom of the shoe to permit pain-free gait.

OTHER SITES OF OSTEOARTHRITIS IN THE FOOT

Osteoarthritis may sometimes occur at the fifth MTP joint, and a bunion at this site is usually attributable to excessively tight shoes (Fig. 6.12). A tracing of the shoe superimposed upon a tracing of the patient's foot will demonstrate that the shoe is indeed smaller than the foot, and the patient should be advised to purchase more comfortable footwear in order to avoid osteoarthritis of the forefoot.

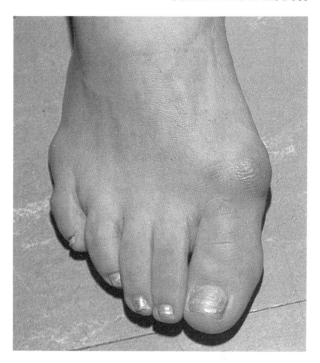

Figure 6.11 In osteoarthritis of the first MTP joint, the bursa between the first metatarsal joint and the skin may become irritated, swollen, and inflamed, giving the characteristic appearance of a bunion (as seen in this photograph).

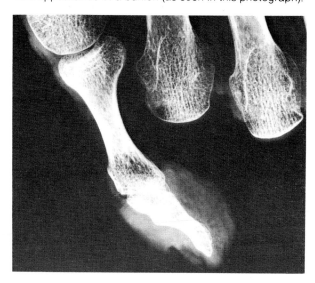

Figure 6.12 Radiograph of the fifth digit of the foot shows medial deviation of the phalanx on the metatarsal bone, and osteophyte formation on the lateral aspect of the metatarsal head.

An anatomic malformation of the foot such as hallux valgus may also lead to degenerative changes in other MTP joints by altering the distribution of mechanical stress. In the clawfoot deformity, chronic hyperextension of the MTP joints results in degenerative changes in the cartilage of the abnormally exposed portion of those joints (Fig. 6.13).

On rare occasions, osteoarthritis may occur in joints other than the MTP. If a patient presents with pain and clinical evidence of osteo-

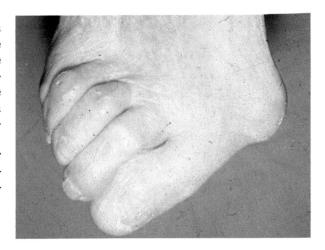

Figure 6.13   In advanced osteoarthritis there may be subluxation of the first phalanx medially, and deformity and enlargement of the head of the first metatarsal bone. This will result in a clawfoot deformity, as seen in the third and fourth toes. The marked hyperextension at the MTP joint and flexion at the PIP joint lead to osteoarthritis in the MTP joint.

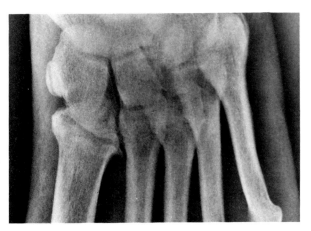

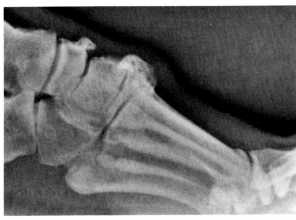

Figure 6.14   Anteroposterior (*left*) and lateral (*right*) radiographs of the foot show extensive osteophyte formation at the first tarsometatarsal joint. This is the most common site of osteoarthritis involving a tarsal bone.

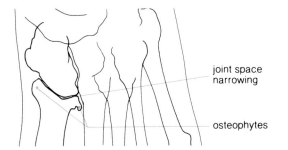

joint space
narrowing

osteophytes

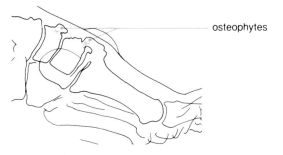

osteophytes

phyte formation over the dorsum of the foot, a radiograph will usually confirm diagnosis of tarsal joint osteoarthritis (Fig. 6.14). Another infrequent site is the talonavicular joint (Fig. 6.15).

The ankle is a particularly unusual site of osteoarthritis, but when it does occur, it is usually secondary to trauma, osteonecrosis, or another mechanical disruption of the joint. Once again, radiographic examination will confirm the diagnosis (Fig. 6.16).

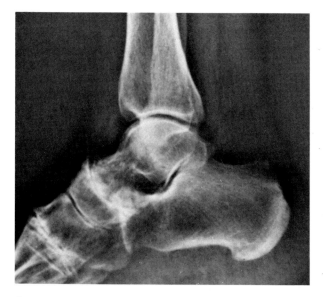

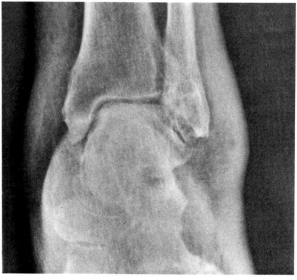

Figure 6.15 Lateral radiograph of the foot demonstrates osteoarthritis of the talonavicular joint, with characteristic joint space narrowing, para-articular sclerosis, and osteophyte formation.

Figure 6.16 Anteroposterior radiograph of the ankle shows joint space narrowing at the fibulotalar aspect, with osteophyte formation and subchondral sclerosis also in evidence, probably secondary to old trauma.

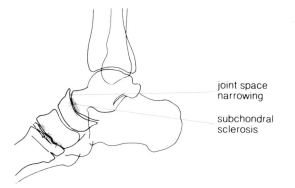

joint space narrowing

subchondral sclerosis

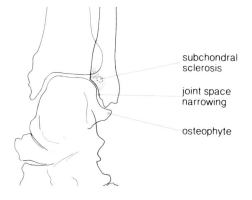

subchondral sclerosis

joint space narrowing

osteophyte

7
Osteoarthritis of the Cervical Spine

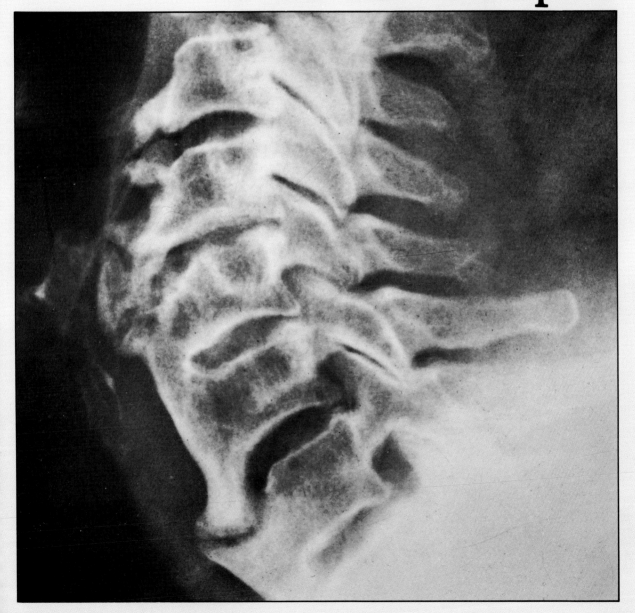

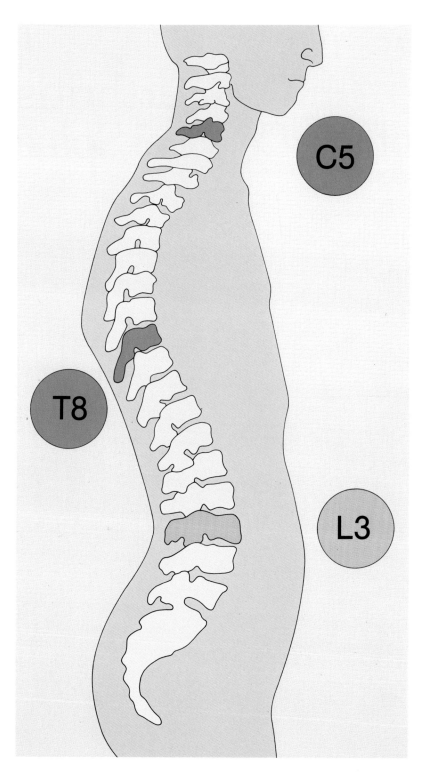

Figure 7.1 In this schematic lateral view of the axial skeleton, cervical and lumbar lordosis and thoracic kyphosis are apparent. Degenerative changes, especially osteophyte formation, occur at the points of greatest concavity which are farthest away from the center of gravity, namely C5, T8, and L3.

The axial skeleton, or spine, is commonly a site for osteoarthritis development. Degenerative changes are seen most frequently in the areas of maximal lordosis or kyphosis, namely C5, T8, and L3–L4. These sites are farthest from the body's center of gravity (Fig. 7.1), and since they are areas of maximal spinal motion, they are more susceptible to wear and tear. Virtually everyone shows some radiographic evidence of osteoarthritis of the spine by age 70.

Although osteoarthritis of the thoracic spine may be extensive, it is usually asymptomatic and represents an incidental finding on chest radiographs. However, the cervical and lumbar spines have been found to be frequent sites for clinically significant osteoarthritis. The lumbar spine will be discussed in Chapter 8. In the cervical spine, degenerative disease may occur at the level of the intervertebral disk, the paired posterior articulations (apophyseal joints), or at the false uncovertebral joints of Luschka (Fig. 7.2).

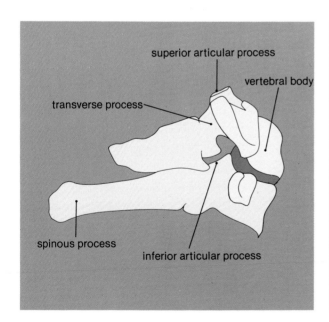

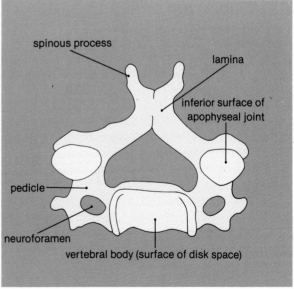

Figure 7.2   Anatomic considerations in degenerative joint disease of the cervical spine. The diagram at left shows a lateral view of two contiguous cervical vertebrae forming the lower functional subunit of the cervical spine. At right is a superior view of a typical cervical vertebra.

ANATOMIC CONSIDERATIONS

Knowledge of the anatomy of the cervical spine is essential to understand the pathophysiologic dynamics of cervical osteoarthritis. The cervical spine is composed of two functional segments. The upper segment consists of the occipitoatlantoid (the skull and C1) and the atlantoaxial (C1–C2) articulations. The first two cervical vertebrae—C1 or *atlas*, and C2 or *axis*—have no posterior articulations, and there are no intervertebral foramina through which the cervical nerves course. The greatest movement found in the cervical spine occurs between C1 and C2 as the atlas rotates around the odontoid process. Indeed, 50 percent of total neck rotation occurs between C1 and C2 before any rotation is noted in the remainder of the cervical spine (Fig. 7.3).

The second segment consists of similar functional subunits in which the anterior aspect serves a weight-bearing, shock-absorbing function and the posterior aspect serves a guiding-gliding function (see Fig. 7.2, *left*). In the anterior aspect of the functional subunit, the disk is a self-contained, fluid-elastic system that absorbs shock, permits transient compression, allows fluid displacement, and accounts for the major movement of the entire cervical spine. The anterior vertical height of the disk is greater than the posterior height. Viewed from the side, the disk is wedge-shaped, a shape which increases the lordotic curvature of the cervical spine (Fig. 7.4). Muscle spasm associated with neck pain, irrespective of underlying cause, may result in considerable loss of lordotic curvature (Fig. 7.5).

In addition to the disk space, the anterior portion of the functional subunit has two lateral, paired articulations known under various names: uncovertebral joints, intervertebral

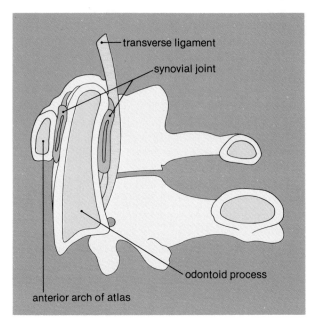

Figure 7.3 This schematic lateral view through a longitudinal section of C1 and C2 demonstrates the intimate relationship as C1 actually encircles the odontoid process of C2. Fifty percent of neck rotation occurs at this location.

articulations, lateral interbody joints, or the joints of Luschka. These are actually bony projections lacking a synovial membrane that articulate to form false joints, or pseudoarthroses. Because these joints do not contain cartilage, they do not develop true osteoarthritis. However, the proliferation of bony projections at this site contributes significantly to the symptomatology of neck pain and cervical radiculitis.

The posterior portion of the functional subunit is composed of two vertebral arches, two transverse processes, a central posterior spinous process, and paired articulations. The posterior articulations, or facets, are true joints containing cartilage capable of undergoing degenerative changes.

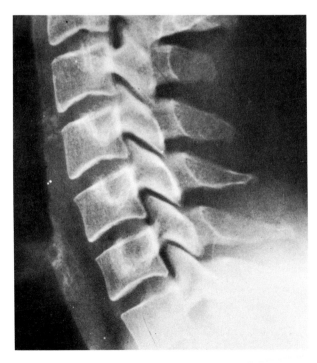

Figure 7.4 Lateral radiograph of a normal cervical spine demonstrates the wedge shape of the cervical disks, a shape which serves to increase the lordosis of the cervical spine. The left and right apophyseal joints can be seen overlapping each other. It should also be noted that each disk space and each vertebra is larger than the one superior to it.

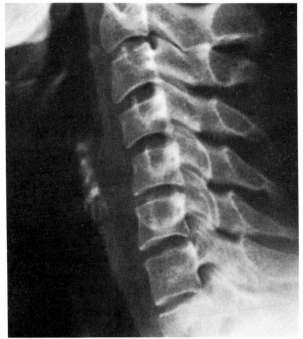

Figure 7.5 Lateral radiograph of the cervical spine reveals a marked straightening, with loss of the normal cervical lordosis secondary to muscle spasm.

The normal physiologic relationship of space to motion in the cervical spine must be understood in order to appreciate cervical dysfunction.

In examining the cervical spine, there are three fields of motion which must be tested: flexion-extension, rotation, and lateral bending (Fig. 7.6). The patient should be able to flex

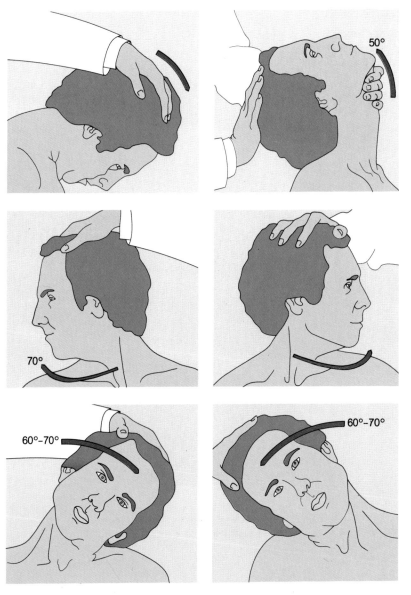

Figure 7.6 Fields of motion in the cervical spine. Flexion-extension (*top*): The patient should be able to flex the neck so that the chin touches the chest wall, and to extend the neck approximately 50°. Rotation (*center*): The patient should be able to rotate the neck 70° to the left and to the right. Lateral bending (*bottom*): The patient should be able to laterally bend the neck 60° to 70°.

the neck so that the chin touches the chest, and to extend the neck approximately 50°. The subject should also be able to rotate the neck 70° to the left and to the right. Lateral bending, the most sensitive aspect of the examination, should be 60° to 70°.

Maximum flexion-extension occurs in the region of C4–C8; consequently, this area has the greatest amount of wear and tear. The neuroforamina close on the side toward which the head bends, and they open on the opposite side (Fig. 7.7). In a normal spine, the degree of narrowing of the foramen is not enough to compress the nerve within the foramen. However, in situations where there is partial bony encroachment upon the neuroforamina, movement may result in further encroachment and cause irritation to the cervical nerve root.

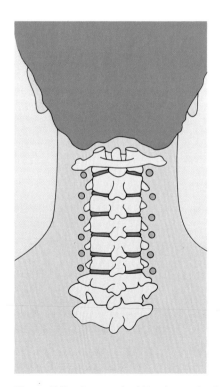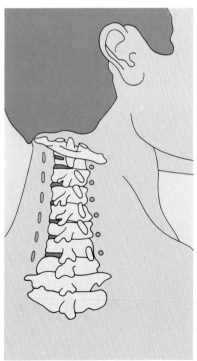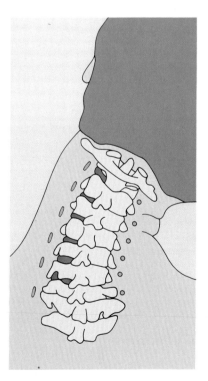

Figure 7.7 As seen in this schematic diagram, the neuroforamina (represented by green dots) close on the side toward which the head rotates or laterally bends, and they open on the opposite side.

CLINICAL FEATURES

The symptoms of cervical osteoarthritis are localized neck pain, stiffness, and the radicular pain radiating down the arm in a dermatomal pattern. These symptoms are brought about by pressure from osteophytes or a prolapsed disk on the spinal roots, spinal cord, or the vertebral artery. Local pain is thought to result from reactions occurring in certain soft

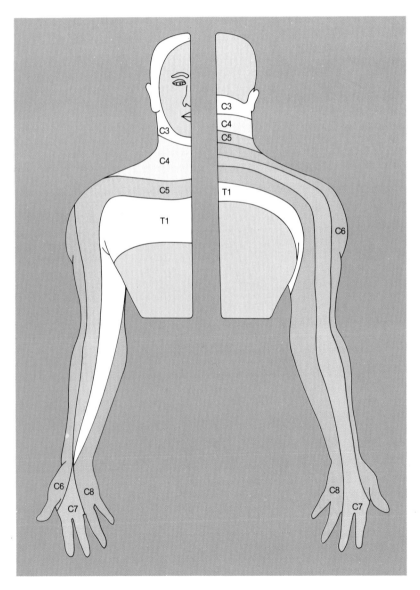

Figure 7.8 Dermatomal distribution in the neck and arm.

tissues, such as the paraspinal ligaments, the joint capsule, and the periosteum, which might explain the spontaneous remissions and exacerbations of symptoms in the presence of persistent or progressive radiologic changes.

Radicular pain is usually associated with the compression of nerve roots, representing referred pain along the associated dermatomes (Fig. 7.8). The localization of arm pain may be helpful in identifying the site of nerve root compression. Classic radicular pain may also be accompanied by paresthesia. In severe cases, patients develop shoulder-hand syndrome (reflex sympathetic dystrophy), with marked swelling of the hand, sweating, and loss of sympathetic tone.

Patients with spinal cord compression usually present with motor weakness in one or both legs associated with paresthesia of the upper extremities. The typical clinical findings consist of an upper motor neuron lesion in one or both lower limbs, coupled with a lower motor neuron lesion in the arms. Myelography should be performed to confirm the level of involvement prior to surgical intervention.

Patients with vertebral artery compression may present with dizziness only; if there is brainstem ischemia, they may also manifest vertigo, tinnitus, diplopia, dysarthria, or dysphagia. Occasionally, patients may experience sudden loss of postural tone or "drop" attacks without loss of consciousness. If symptoms are exacerbated by rotation or flexion of the neck, a cervical collar may be useful. In rare cases, angiographic studies of the vertebral arteries may be necessary to determine the degree of atheromatous narrowing of the vessel and the extent of encroachment by the osteophyte. If the primary problem is encroachment, surgical decompression may be warranted.

Many conditions simulate pain in the neck or shoulder and feelings of discomfort or dysesthesia in the upper extremity that must be differentiated from cervical osteoarthritis (Table 7.1).

Table 7.1 Differential Diagnosis of Neck Pain

Degenerative Changes
Degenerative disk disease
Herniated cervical disk
Apophyseal osteoarthritis
Uncovertebral joint degeneration

Inflammatory or Infectious Diseases
Rheumatoid arthritis (especially C1–C2)
Ankylosing spondylitis
Septic spondylitis
Osteomyelitis

Metabolic Disorders
Osteoporosis with vertebral collapse
Paget's disease

Neoplasms
Primary or metastatic tumors
Pancoast's tumor

Cervical Neurovascular Syndromes
Cervical rib
Scalene muscle
Rib clavicle compression
Hyperabductor syndrome

Miscellaneous Disorders
Torticollis
Cervical lymphadenitis
Muscle strain
Reflex sympathetic dystrophy

Pathologic Considerations

The symptoms of cervical osteoarthritis occur as a consequence of cervical disk disease, osteophyte formation at the uncovertebral joints, and/or apophyseal joint degeneration.

Cervical Disk Disease

Whereas acute protrusion of the cervical disk is a relatively uncommon cause of cervical radiculopathy, disk degeneration is frequently found to be responsible for manifestations such as neck pain, nerve root pathology, and spinal cord compression. Ultimately, all disks undergo some degree of degenerative change, which may result from nuclear herniation, annular protrusion, or dehydration and fissuring of disk material. Pathologically, this is seen as a decrease in the height of the disk space in conjunction with, or without, osteophyte formation (Fig. 7.9).

With increasing fragmentation, the nuclear material bulges outward through the rents in the annulus. This sequence continues until the nuclear material is both against and held by the longitudinal ligament. As the disk degenerates, the intradisk pressure decreases, the

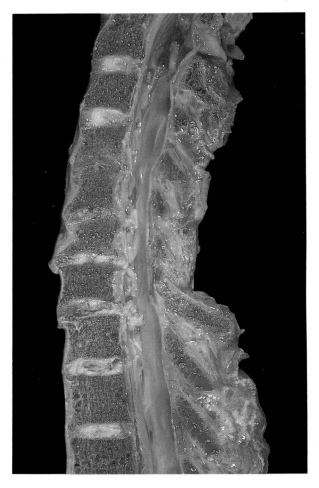

Figure 7.9 Gross sagittal section of the cervical spine reveals severe disk degeneration at C3–C4, C4–C5, and C5–C6, marked by a decrease in the height of the disk spaces at these locations. Anterior osteophytes are in evidence at C5–C6.

annulus bulges, and the vertebral end plates approximate. The most common site for intervertebral disk collapse is C5–C6, with C4–C5 and C6–C7 being equally affected thereafter (Fig. 7.10).

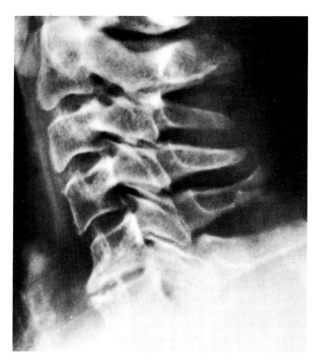 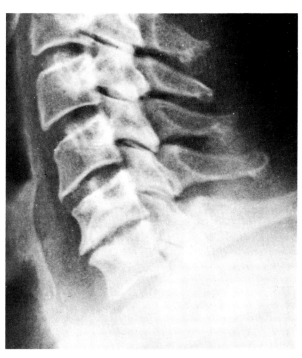

Figure 7.10 Cervical disk disease can be most readily observed on lateral radiographs of the cervical spine. In the radiograph at left one may observe disk space narrowing and osteophyte formation anteriorly at C5–C6, the most common site of degenerative disk disease. As seen in the radiograph at right, similar findings may occasionally be observed at C6–C7. A single disk may be involved, or in more advanced disease, multiple disks may show degeneration.

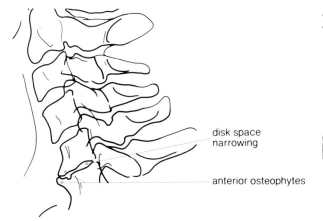

disk space narrowing

anterior osteophytes

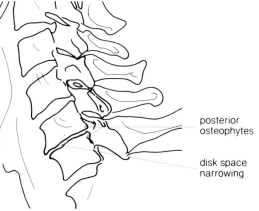

posterior osteophytes

disk space narrowing

Narrowing of the disk space can be more easily noted on lateral radiographic view, but may also be observed on anteroposterior view (Fig. 7.11). Disk collapse may also occur at other interspaces, but this finding should suggest either old trauma or rheumatoid arthritis (Fig. 7.12). Disk fragmentation may lead to subluxation of one vertebra on another, with the development of secondary osteoarthritis of the facet joints (Fig. 7.13).

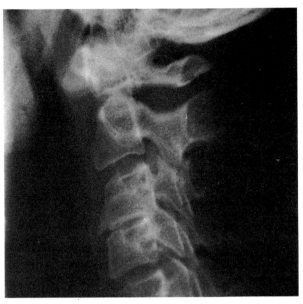

Figure 7.12   Lateral radiograph of the cervical spine shows marked disk space narrowing at C3–C4, which should suggest the diagnosis of old trauma or rheumatoid arthritis. Note also the marked loss of cervical lordosis.

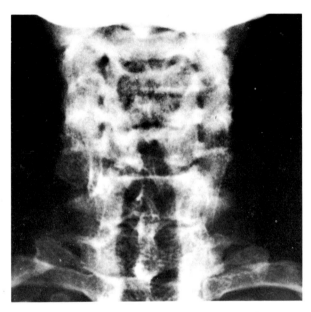

Figure 7.11   Anteroposterior radiograph shows marked narrowing of the disk spaces at C2–C3 and C3–C4, especially when compared to the relatively normal height of the disk space at C4–C5.

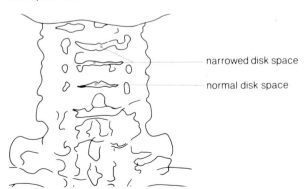

narrowed disk space

normal disk space

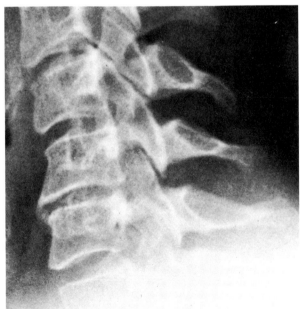

Figure 7.13   In advanced cervical osteoarthritis, subluxation of the vertebrae may occur. In this lateral radiograph, C4 is subluxed on C5, and disk collapse at C5–C6 is evident.

Osteophyte Formation

As the disk continues to degenerate and approximation of the two adjacent vertebrae occurs, the usually taut posterior longitudinal ligament begins to slacken and is dissected away from the periosteum by extruding disk material. Osteophytes may form at these sites of periosteal injury as extruded disk material becomes fibrosed and calcified.

Anterior osteophytes are frequently noted, but due to their location, they are usually asymptomatic (Fig. 7.14). In patients with ankylosing hyperostosis (Forrestiere's disease), the abundant osteophyte formation may be so extensive that it partially obstructs the esophagus, causing the patient to complain of a sticking sensation in the throat, i.e., dysphagia (Fig. 7.15).

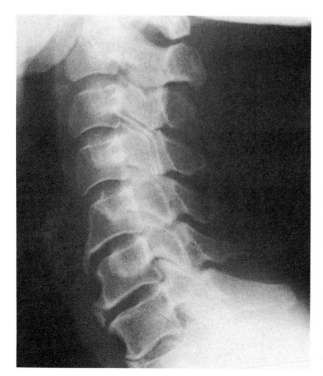

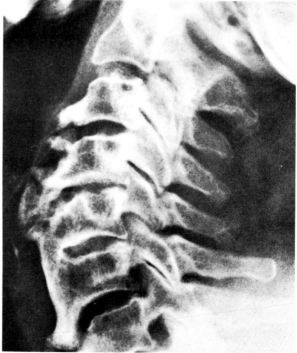

Figure 7.14 Lateral radiograph of the cervical spine reveals anterior osteophytes at the margins of C5, C6, and C7. These osteophytes are usually asymptomatic.

Figure 7.15 Lateral radiograph of the cervical spine in a patient with ankylosing hyperostosis reveals exuberant anterior osteophyte formation.

The approximation of the vertebral bodies also approximates the uncovertebral joints of Luschka, and with constant irritation and friction they also become the sites of osteophyte formation (Fig. 7.16). Degenerative changes in the cervical spine that evolve from disk degeneration deform the intervertebral foramina as well as change the size and shape of the spinal canal. In oblique radiographs of the cervical spine, the uncovertebral joint is seen at

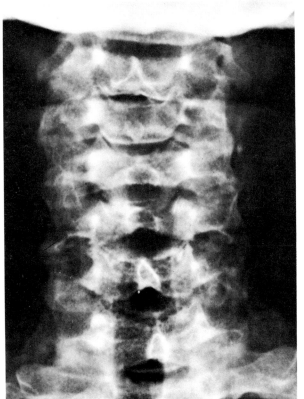

Figure 7.16 Anteroposterior radiograph of the cervical spine shows posterior osteophyte formation at the uncovertebral joint. Early new bone formation can also be noted at C5–C6 on the right.

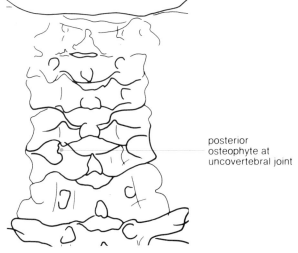

posterior osteophyte at uncovertebral joint

the inferior medial aspect of the neurofora-
men, causing nerve root irritation or compression (Fig. 7.17). Radicular symptoms only
manifest with 50 to 75 percent osteophytic
encroachment.

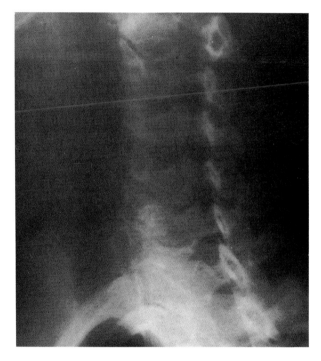 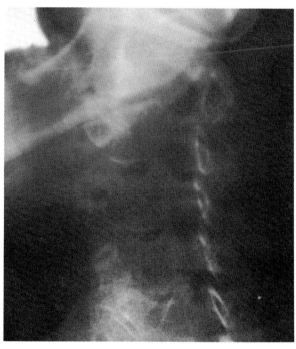

Figure 7.17 The neuroforamina and the uncovertebral joints can be best observed on oblique radiographs. At left, the neuroforaminal openings are shown increasing in size from C1 to C7. Since the nerve root rests on the floor of the neuroforamina, small osteophytes may occasionally bring about radicular symptoms. At right, osteophytes can be seen on the superior medial aspect of the C5–C6 neurofora-men, decreasing the diameter of the foramen.

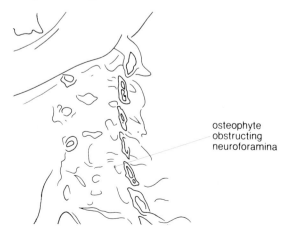

osteophyte
obstructing
neuroforamina

Apophyseal Joint Degeneration

The approximation of the anterior components of the functional units inevitably results in degenerative changes in the apophyseal or facet joint. Radiographically, the usual joint space narrowing, para-articular sclerosis, osteophyte formation, and loss of cartilage are evident (Fig. 7.18). Ultimately, encroachment from the posterior inferior margin into the intervertebral foramen occurs.

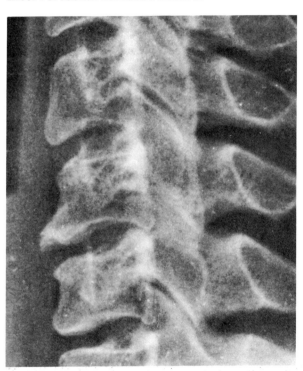

Figure 7.18   Lateral radiograph of the cervical spine shows slight disk space narrowing at C5 and C6, as well as apophyseal joint degeneration. Since the apophyseal joint is a true diarthrodial joint, the osteoarthritic manifestations are the same as seen elsewhere: nonuniform joint space narrowing, osteophyte formation, and para-articular sclerosis.

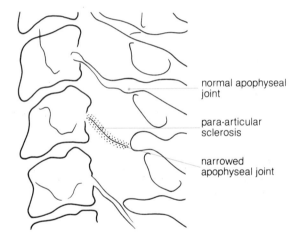

normal apophyseal joint

para-articular sclerosis

narrowed apophyseal joint

8
Osteoarthritis of the Lumbar Spine

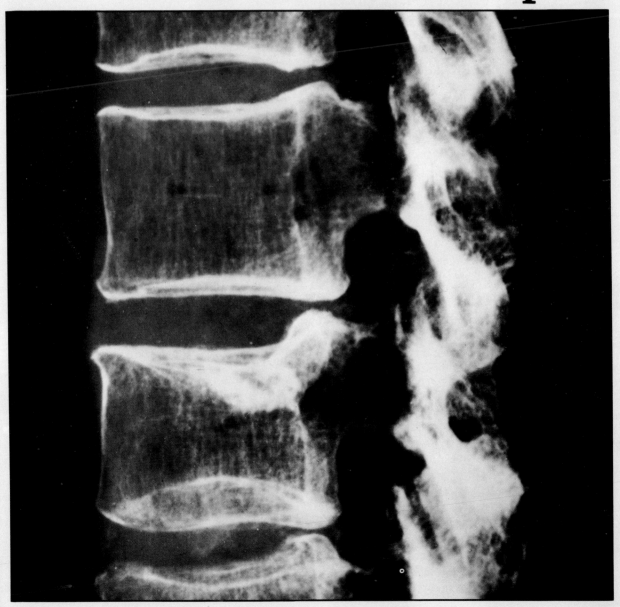

Low back pain is one of the most common conditions seen by medical practitioners, and is a major cause of disability. The most common identifiable cause of low back pain is osteoarthritis of the lumbar spine. The posterior apophyseal joints are true diarthrodial joints, and therefore may undergo the typical changes of osteoarthritis. The degenerative changes that occur in the anterior or intervertebral disk unit are more accurately referred to as spondylosis.

ANATOMIC CONSIDERATIONS

The low back region is defined as the area of the spine below the L1 level. The lumbar spine comprises L1 through L5 and has a functional subunit, the anterior and posterior portions of which perform different but essential roles (Fig. 8.1). The anterior portion consists of two

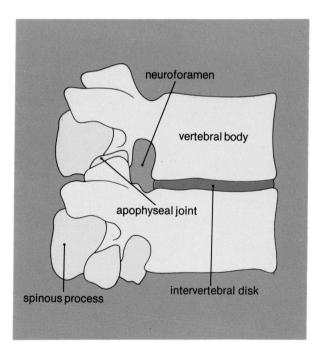

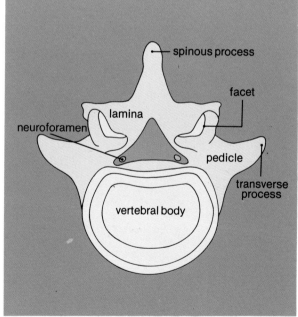

Figure 8.1 Schematic lateral view of the lumbar spine (*left*) reveals that the functional subunit consists of two portions. The anterior portion, consisting of vertebral bodies and an intervertebral disk, functions in weight bearing. The posterior portion is involved in the gliding-guiding function of the lumbar spine. On superior view (*right*), the posterior portion, consisting of the lamina, pedicles, and facets, is clearly seen. The apophyseal (facet) joints serve as the posterior wall of the neuroforamina.

cylindrical vertebral bodies separated by a hydraulic system called the disk. The disk is a self-contained fluid system that absorbs shock, permits transient compression, and allows for movement. The posterior portion is composed of two vertebral arches, two transverse processes, a central spinous process, and paired articulations called facets. In the lumbar region, the facets lie in the vertical sagittal plane, thus permitting flexion and extension of the region (Fig. 8.2). In the thoracic spine, the facets lie in a horizontal plane, which allows for side bending and rotation about a vertical line. The facet joint serves as a guiding mechanism without any weight-bearing function.

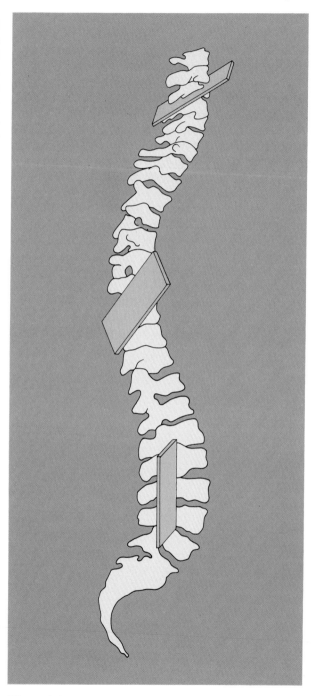

Figure 8.2 Schematic diagram illustrates the orientation of the facet joints in the various regions of the spine. In the lumbar region, the facets are in the vertical sagittal plane, permitting flexion and extension.

Experimental evidence suggests that low back pain originates from one of the following sources: (1) irritation of the posterior longitudinal ligament by increasing the interdisk pressure in a previously degenerated disk, (2) a synovitis of the articular facets with resultant periarticular muscle spasm (limitation of motion may be progressive), (3) the concomitant muscle spasm that accompanies spinal dysfunction, and (4) irritation of the nerve root as it passes through the intervertebral foramen.

In the vast majority of painful states, an increase in the lumbosacral angle results in an accentuation of the lumbar lordosis, a condition termed "swayback" (Fig. 8.3). Probably 75 percent of all postural low back pain can be attributed to an exaggerated lumbar lordosis.

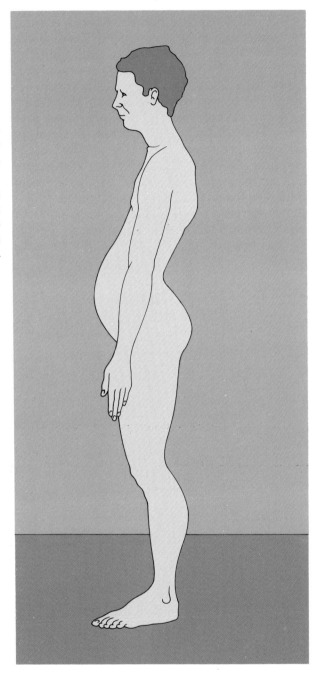

Figure 8.3   A poor posture and musculoskeletal condition may lead to a protruding abdomen, the appearance of being overweight, and an exaggerated lumbar lordosis ("swayback"). Poor muscle tone is secondary to a lack of regular exercise.

Pathologic Considerations

Aging decreases the elastic properties of the intervertebral disk. In young patients, the nucleus pulposus is 80 percent water. As the nucleus pulposus ages it loses its water-binding capacity, and the collagenous rings that encase the disk become fragmented. Brief compressive loads imposed upon a normal disk may cause distortion, but no permanent deformity (Fig. 8.4). However, constant pressure on the disk, whether sustained or recurrent, plays a substantial role in the degeneration of the unit. Spondylosis is a sequela of intervertebral disk degeneration, and pain may occur by one of several mechanisms.

As the vertebrae approximate, the ligaments slacken and may be dissected away from their periosteal attachments by extruded disk material. The extrusion of disk material further decreases the quantity of disk material between the vertebrae, and a vicious cycle is established. The extruded material then evokes a local reaction that is subsequently replaced with fibrous tissue calcification and/or ossification (Fig. 8.5),

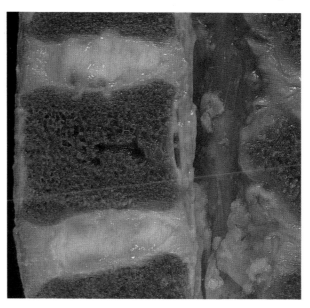

Figure 8.4 Gross sagittal section of the lumbar spine of a 40-year-old subject shows that there is good preservation of the disk height and no evidence of osteophyte formation.

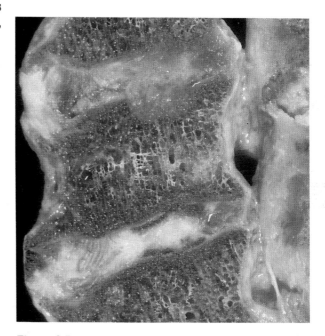

Figure 8.5 Gross sagittal section of the lumbar spine shows markedly narrowed disk spaces, marked anterior herniation at L4–L5 and L5–S1, and significant osteophyte formation.

and ultimately this will be seen radiographically as an osteophytic spur (Figs. 8.6 and 8.7).

Narrowing of the anterior functional unit by disk collapse results in approximation of the facet joint, with subsequent facet malalign-

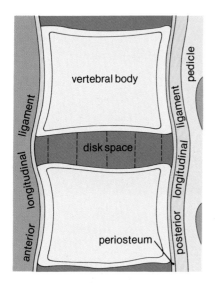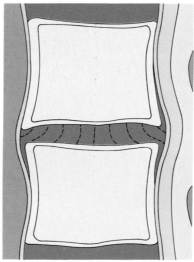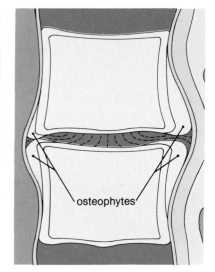

Figure 8.6 Schematic diagrams illustrate vertebral disk degeneration. Under normal conditions, the posterior longitudinal ligament is loosely adherent to the vertebral body periosteum (*left*). Disk degeneration causes approximation of the two vertebrae, resulting in slackening of the ligament and permitting dissection between the periosteum and the ligament (*center*). Subsequently, extruded disk material becomes ossified into osteophytic spurs (*right*).

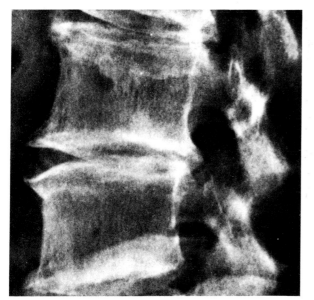

Figure 8.7 In this lateral radiograph, both anterior and posterior vertebral osteophytes are evident at L3 and L4. Anterior osteophytes, in and of themselves, are rarely the cause of clinically significant symptoms related to the back.

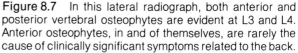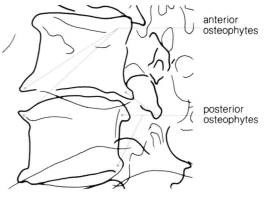

ment and, ultimately, encroachment upon the intervertebral foramina (Fig. 8.8). This encroachment arises because of the approximation of the two pedicles: anteriorly by the bulging of the longitudinal ligament and (possibly) early spur formation, and posteriorly by the encroaching facets. Hyperextension of the lumbar spine may further aggravate the nerve root and mimic the clinical pattern of pain (Fig. 8.9). Neurogenic claudication may be evident if lateral stenosis occurs.

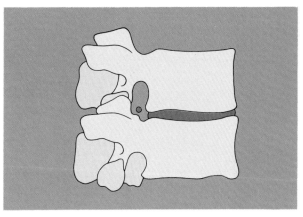

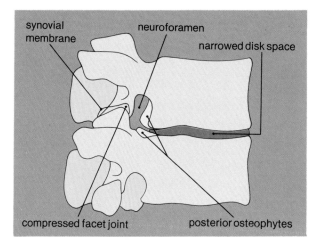

Figure 8.8 This diagram demonstrates foraminal narrowing due to osteophyte impingement, and posterior articular compression by the encroaching facets.

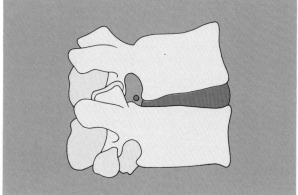

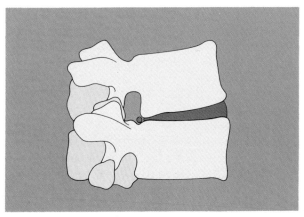

Figure 8.9 In a normal disk (*top*), hyperextension of the vertebral segment can mechanically irritate the nerve root and cause pain by compression of the nerve (*center*). This is much more likely to occur when the increased angulation is combined with a narrowed disk space, a consequence of lumbar disk disease (*bottom*).

Another aspect of lumbar disk disease is disk rupture (herniation), during which nuclear material is suddenly released from the capsule. When the protrusion is posterolateral, acute nerve root compression results (Fig. 8.10). A centromedial protrusion may cause cauda equina compression with resultant anesthesia in a saddle distribution. Motor weakness may be profound, and both ankle reflexes may be lost. Acute urinary retention can occur in association with cauda equina compression, and is an indication for emergency myelography and surgery.

CLINICAL FEATURES OF LOW BACK PAIN SYNDROME

The patient with lumbar disk disease presents with a clinical history of pain in the lower back or buttocks that radiates down the leg (sciatica). Although a history of trauma, heavy lifting, or hearing a "snap" in the back may occasionally be obtained in patients with an acutely herniated disk, the relationship between stress and the onset of pain is rather infrequent. Sciatic pain is usually referred to the posterior thigh, the calf, the heel, and into the toes. The initial pain may be described as sharp or dull, continuous or intermittent. Numbness of the leg may precede or accompany the pain. The localization of numbness may be an important aspect in identifying the site of the arthritis.

Nerve root irritation may cause radiation of the pain into the hip region with no distal radiation, and may be mistaken for hip joint arthritis. The presence of a full range of pain-free hip motions and a negative Laségue's sign should confirm the site of disease as the back.

Pressure exerted upon an irritable nerve is sufficient to cause pain. Standing or sitting, which increases intradisk pressure and causes further disk bulging, can aggravate sciatica. The intradisk pressure in a supine person is 30 percent less than the pressure standing, and 50 percent less than the pressure sitting. The pressure within a lumbar disk is thus greatest

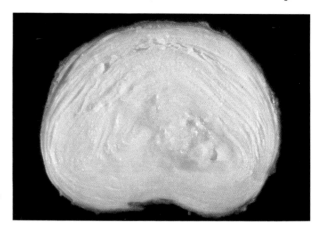

Figure 8.10   Cross-section of a lumbar disk shows protrusion of nuclear material into the posterolateral aspect of the annulus.

during sitting and least when reclining, and these findings may explain the relief of symptoms when a patient assumes complete bed rest.

Tests for Low Back Pain Syndrome

In examining an individual with low back pain syndrome, the standing posture must be evaluated. Lumbar spasm usually causes a flattening of the lordotic curvature and lateral scoliosis. (Lateral scoliosis of the spine is frequently to the side of the nerve root irritation.) Spasm may be detected when the patient attempts to bend forward. A persistence of the lumbar lordotic curve while bending forward indicates the limitation of functional motion in the lumbar area (Fig. 8.11). The limitation of lateral motion is not useful from a diagnostic point of view.

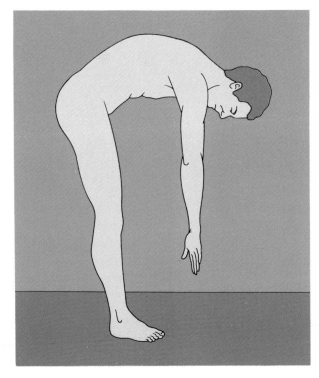
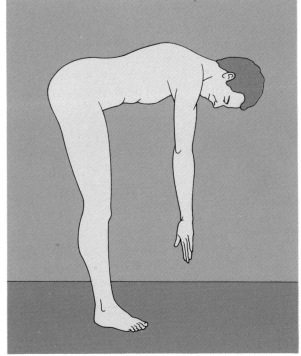

Figure 8.11   Normally, on flexion of the lumbar spine, the lumbar lordosis is completely lost, and the spinal column has a smooth, curved contour when viewed from the side (*left*). Persistence of lumbar lordosis while flexing (*right*) indicates limitation of motion in the lumbar vertebrae, and is usually associated with spasm of the paravertebral muscles.

The straight leg raising test is performed with the patient in the supine position (Fig. 8.12). The leg is elevated with the knee extended. During the first 15° to 30° of elevation, there is no movement of the nerve roots at the neuroforamina. When the leg reaches an angle of 30°, traction on the sciatic nerve occurs, followed by downward movement of the roots in their foramina. The greatest degree of movement occurs in the L5 root. In a positive test,

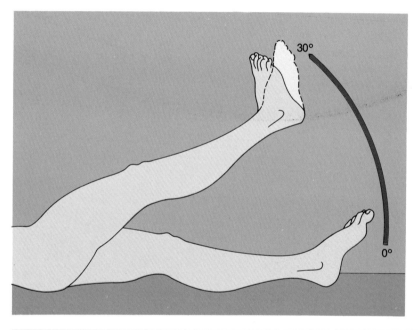

Figure 8.12 In the straight leg raising test, the leg is elevated with the knee extended. At 30° of elevation, the patient may experience pain in the low back area or in the thigh. Dorsiflexion of the foot at this point exacerbates the sensation of pain in the low back or thigh.

Table 8.1 Level and Neurologic Effect of Nerve Root Impingement

Level of Disease	Root Involved	Straight Leg Raising Test	Deep-Tendon Reflexes	Muscles Showing Weakness
L2–L3	L3	Negative	Normal	Quadriceps femoris
L3–L4	L4	Negative	Loss of knee reflex	Quadriceps femoris
L4–L5	L5	Positive	Normal	
L5–S1	S1	Positive	Loss of ankle reflex	Gastrocnemius and soleus

the patient experiences pain in the low back area or in the thigh when the leg is elevated above 30°. If the foot is forcefully dorsiflexed while the leg is held at 15° to 30°, pain may be exacerbated. A positive test localizes disk disease to the L5–S1 or L4–L5 level, but the test will not detect disk disease at higher interspaces.

A thorough neurologic examination can confirm the level of nerve root irritation (Table 8.1). A pin-prick test can be used to map out areas of hypalgesia or numbness, and the use of a standard dermatomal map (Fig. 8.13) can be used to identify the involved nerve root. Deep-tendon reflexes should be evaluated and compared, relating one side to the other. In patients with nerve root irritation, depression of the reflex on only one side may be evident, or a total loss of the reflex may occur. The ankle reflex is dependent on an intact S1 motor root. A depressed knee reflex represents pressure on the L4 root. The absence of bilateral deep-tendon reflexes at one level is possible in a patient with central disk herniation.

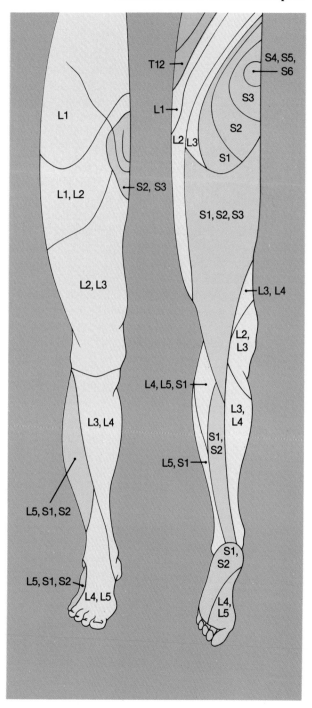

Figure 8.13   This modified dermatomal map demonstrates the levels and locations of pain and numbness associated with lumbar disk disease.

The differential diagnosis of low back pain is quite extensive (Table 8.2). Establishing the diagnosis of those diseases that require specific therapy is of primary importance. The diagnoses of osteomyelitis, neoplastic disease, and metabolic bone disease can usually be made on the basis of radiographs of the lumbar spine.

RADIOGRAPHIC FEATURES OF OSTEOARTHRITIS

Radiographically, the lumbar spine is most easily evaluated on lateral and oblique views. On lateral view, the individual vertebrae and disk spaces are more clearly delineated, with each disk space larger than the one above it. On oblique view, the apophyseal or facet joints are best demonstrated.

Lumbar disk disease or spondylosis can usually be diagnosed on a lateral radiograph by noting a narrowing of the disk space. As previously noted, L4–L5 is the most frequently involved disk space in lumbar disk disease.

Table 8.2 Differential Diagnosis of Low Back Pain

Structural
Herniated intervertebral disk
Spondylosis and apophyseal
 osteoarthritis
Hyperostotic spondylosis
Spinal stenosis
Spondylolisthesis
Fractures
Congenital abnormalities

Inflammatory
Ankylosing spondylitis
Other inflammatory
 spondyloarthropathies
Rheumatoid arthritis
Osteomyelitis

Neoplastic
Primary and metastatic tumors
Multiple myeloma

Metabolic
Hyperparathyroidism
Paget's disease
Ochronosis

Referred pain

The lateral radiographs in Figure 8.14 show progressive narrowing of the L4–L5 disk space over a 7-year period. In addition, adjacent "discogenic sclerosis" of L4 can be noted in both radiographs.

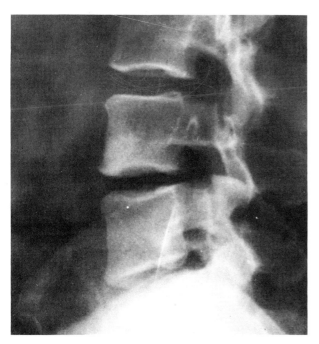
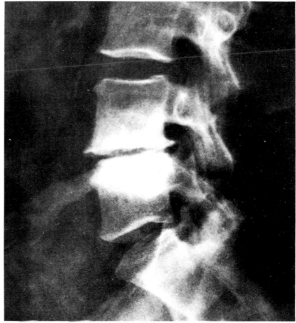

Figure 8.14   Lateral radiograph of the lumbar spine (*left*) shows narrowing of the L4–L5 disk space, which would normally be larger than the L3–L4 space. Sclerosis of the adjacent L4 vertebral body ("discogenic sclerosis") is also apparent. Lateral radiograph of the same patient taken 7 years later (*right*) reveals extensive degeneration of the L4–L5 disk space. In addition, there has been progressive narrowing of the disk space, anterior and posterior osteophyte formation, and increasing discogenic sclerosis of the adjacent vertebral bodies.

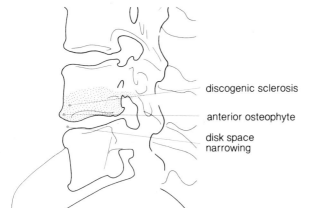
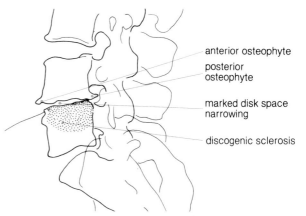

discogenic sclerosis

anterior osteophyte

disk space narrowing

anterior osteophyte

posterior osteophyte

marked disk space narrowing

discogenic sclerosis

In advanced osteoarthritis, there may be many levels of disk space involvement, with marked disk space narrowing involving virtually all of the lumbar disk spaces (Fig. 8.15). When the disk herniates into the adjacent vertebral body, the resulting area of demineralization is known as Schmorl's nodes (Fig. 8.16, *left*). Pathologic observations reveal disk material invaginating into the body of the vertebra (Fig. 8.16, *right*).

On oblique views of the lumbar spine, the apophyseal joints are seen as vertical lucent areas in the middle of the vertebrae. As elsewhere, the characteristic features are loss of joint space and para-articular sclerosis. In the

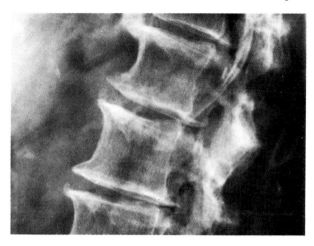

Figure 8.15 Lateral radiograph of the lumbar spine in advanced osteoarthritis reveals extensive disk space degeneration involving virtually all of the lumbar disk spaces.

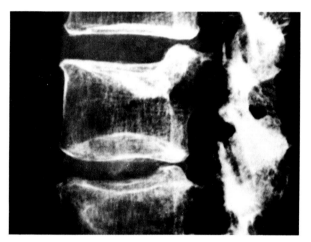

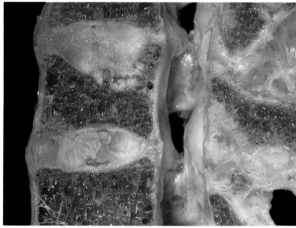

Figure 8.16 Lateral postmortem radiograph (*left*) reveals a herniation of disk material into the posterior aspect of the superior endplate of L2 (Schmorl's node). Reactive sclerosis is also in evidence at the site of the herniation. Gross sagittal section of the same vertebrae (*right*) shows disk material penetrating into the body of L2.

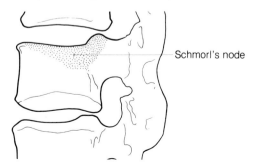

Schmorl's node

radiograph in Figure 8.17, these changes can be noted at the L5–S1 apophyseal articulation. In more advanced disease, the para-articular sclerosis is evident on anteroposterior view and may be mistaken for an osteoblastic lesion. For example, the anteroposterior radiograph in Figure 8.18 (*left*) shows severe para-articular sclerosis and joint space narrowing at the L4–L5 and L5–S1 apophyseal joints bilaterally. An oblique view (Fig. 8.18, *right*) confirms the observation that the sclerosis is localized to the para-articular area, and this finding represents osteoarthritis rather than Paget's disease or an osteoblastic lesion.

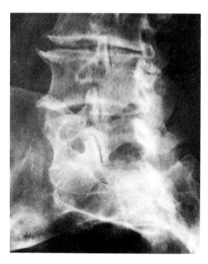

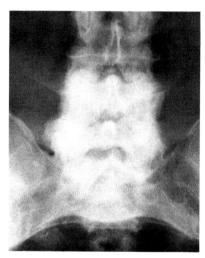

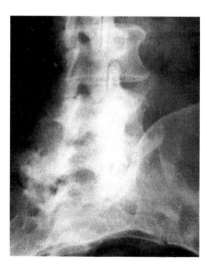

Figure 8.17 Oblique radiograph shows joint space narrowing, osteophyte formation, and bony sclerosis at the L5–S1 apophyseal joint.

Figure 8.18 Anteroposterior radiograph of the lumbar spine (*left*) reveals extensive bony sclerosis which appears to involve L4 and L5 bilaterally.

An oblique radiograph of this spine (*right*) localizes the sclerosis to the apophyseal joint area at L4–L5 and L5–S1.

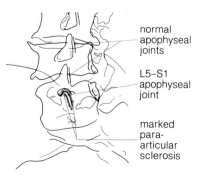

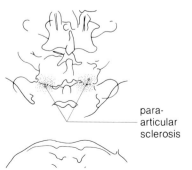

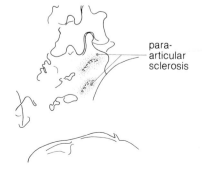

Slippage of the vertebrae (degenerative spondylolisthesis) may occur independently of a break in the pars interarticularis, and is usually associated with advanced osteoarthritis of the apophyseal joints combined with lumbar disk disease (Fig. 8.19). The radiograph in Figure 8.20 shows slippage of L4 on L5 as a result of extensive osteoarthritis of the facet joint.

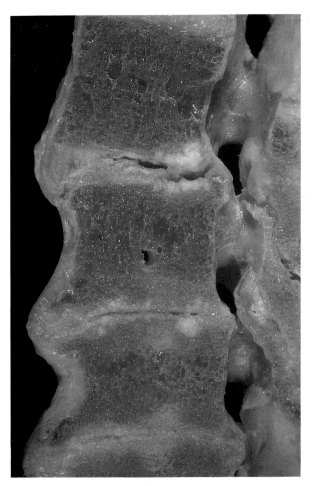

Figure 8.19   Gross sagittal section of the lumbar spine shows anterior slippage of L2 on L3 with cleavage of the disk, characteristic of spondylolisthesis. Note the virtual absence of the L3–L4 and L4–L5 disk spaces.

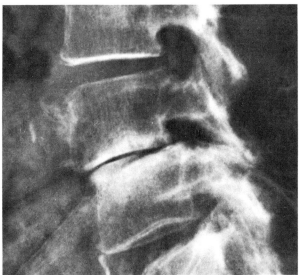

Figure 8.20   Spondylolisthesis: Lateral radiograph shows that the L4 vertebral body has slipped onto L5.

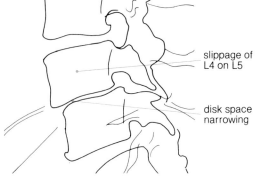

slippage of
L4 on L5

disk space
narrowing

Minor anomalies of the vertebrae are so common that a variation from normal is detectable in about 50 percent of the population. Of these anomalies, only the presence of a sixth lumbar vertebra and sacralization of the fifth lumbar vertebra are clinically important. Sacralization, reduction in the number of mobile vertebrae in the lumbar region to four, is unlikely to cause symptoms when the entire vertebra is solidly incorporated into the sacrum. The most common form of sacralization is for one of the transverse processes of the fifth lumbar vertebra to be enlarged and joined to the sacrum by a diarthrodial joint (Bertolotti's syndrome) (Fig. 8.21). This diarthrodial joint may be subject to abnormal stresses which result in osteoarthritis of the new joint.

In the absence of radiographic evidence of lumbar spine disease, and in a clinical situation in which an acute disk protrusion may be suspected, two investigative tests may be warranted: computed axial tomography (CT scan) and myelography. The former is a noninvasive procedure, and may be of use in reveal-

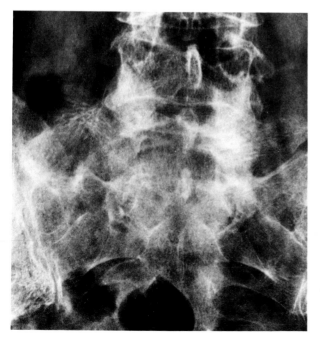

Figure 8.21 In the most common form of sacralization, one of the transverse processes of the fifth lumbar vertebra may be enlarged and joined to the sacrum by a diarthrodial joint. As seen here, narrowing of the joint space and bony sclerosis are indicative of osteoarthritis in this new joint.

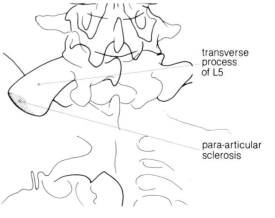

transverse process of L5

para-articular sclerosis

ing the extent of spinal stenosis (Fig. 8.22) and determining acute disk prolapses (Fig. 8.23). The extent of disk space disruption can be demonstrated by injecting radiopaque material in the disk space (a diskogram) (Fig. 8.24). The latter is an invasive technique that

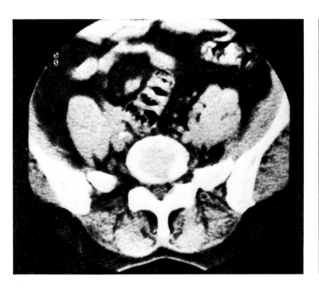 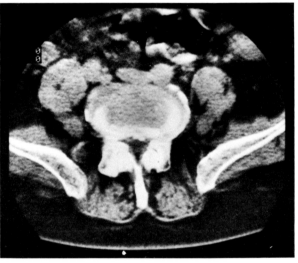

Figure 8.22   In the CT scan at left, the normal spinal canal can be observed between the body of the vertebra and the posterior spinous process. Epidural fat can be seen as radiolucent areas at the apices of the spinal canal. However, in the CT scan at right, one may note marked osteophyte formation at the facet joints, leading to narrowing of the lumbar spinal canal and resulting in spinal stenosis. Note the loss of the epidural fat radiolucencies as osteophytes impinge upon the canal. The radiodense material along the right aspect of the disk represents a large osteophyte.

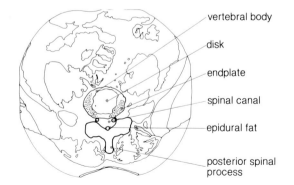 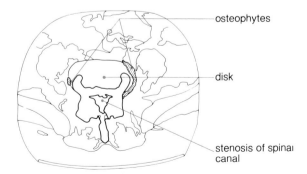

should be limited to those patients in whom surgery is being contemplated, specifically in patients who exhibit neurologic deficits while under observation. In a typical myelogram, the extent and location of the disk protrusion can be accurately demonstrated to facilitate an appropriate surgical procedure.

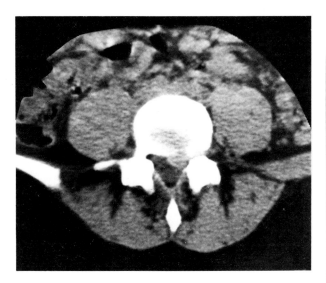

Figure 8.23   This CT scan through the disk space of L5–S1 shows posterior herniation of the nucleus pulposus (predominantly on the left side), which almost certainly was responsible for the left-sided sciatic pain experienced by this patient. (Courtesy of Dr. James G. Hirschy)

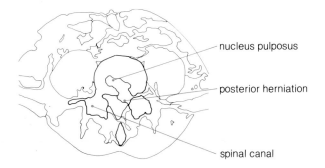

nucleus pulposus

posterior herniation

spinal canal

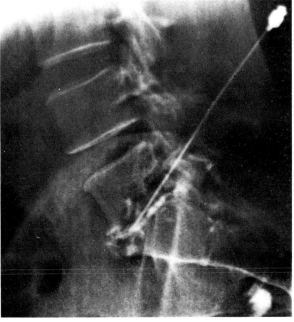

Figure 8.24   Diskogram with radiopaque material injected into the disk space shows protrusion of dye anteriorly and posteriorly, demonstrating herniation of disk material.

In situations where surgery is warranted, a standard lateral radiograph may demonstrate apophyseal as well as disk space narrowing without clearly identifying the extent of encroachment upon the spinal canal and its contents (Fig. 8.25, *left*). The myelogram, on the other hand, will usually demonstrate the degree of encroachment, seen at virtually all lumbar levels in Figure 8.25, *right*.

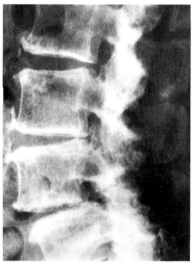 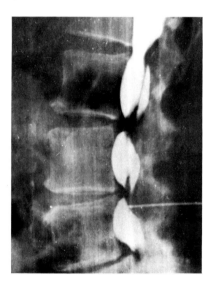

Figure 8.25 Lateral radiograph of the lumbar spine (*left*) shows extensive apophyseal osteoarthritis (identified here primarily as para-articular sclerosis). In addition, there is disk space narrowing at L4–L5 and sublux- ation of L4 on L5. A myelogram of this spine (*right*) reveals anterior as well as posterior encroachment at levels L1–L2, L2–L3, L3–L4, and L4–L5. Such extensive encroachment leads to a functional spinal stenosis.

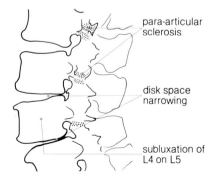 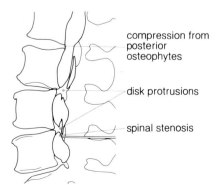

9

Miscellaneous Aspects of Osteoarthritis
Sports-relatedness and Atypical Sites

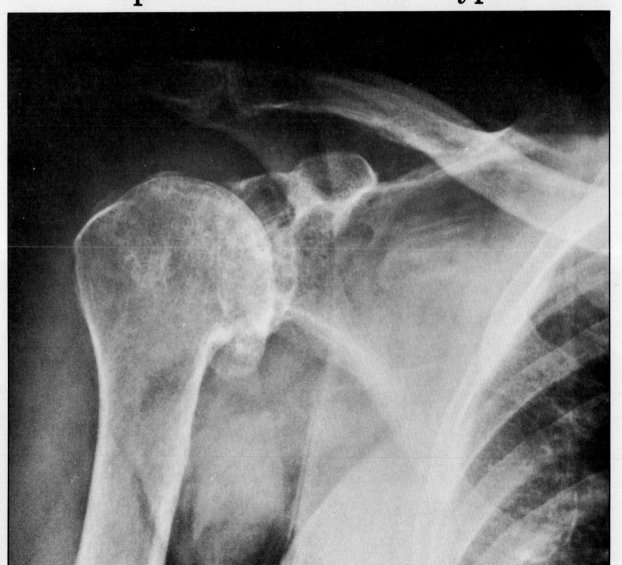

While clinical osteoarthritis is most commonly seen in the joints discussed in earlier chapters, it is by no means limited to those joints. Indeed, osteoarthritis may occur in any diarthrodial joint that is subjected to unusual stresses or functional overloading. The latter is clearly an occupational hazard for those involved in athletics and heavy industry, leading to the subsequent development of clinical disease in unusual sites such as the shoulders (Fig. 9.1), elbows (Fig. 9.2), or wrists (Fig. 9.3) of baseball pitchers and pneumatic drill operators, or in the ankles of basketball players. The current enthusiasm for running as a means of improving cardiovascular fitness, relieving stress, and avoiding obesity has resulted in a much larger population at risk for athletic injuries which might eventuate in osteoarthritis.

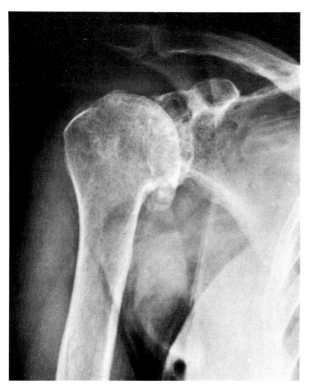

Figure 9.1 Anteroposterior radiograph of the shoulder shows a large osteophyte extending from the inferior margin of the head of the humerus. In addition, one can observe marked subchondral bony sclerosis as well as irregularity in the contour of the head of the humerus.

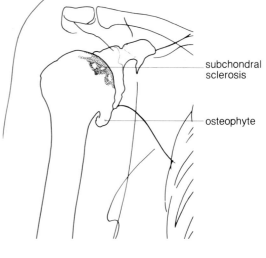

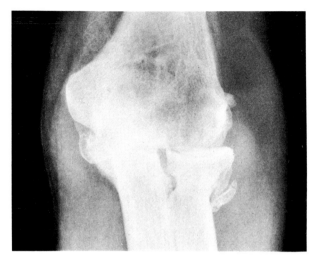

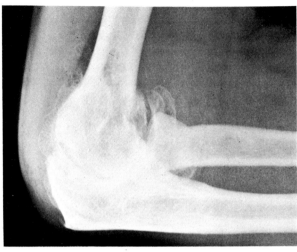

Figure 9.2 Anteroposterior radiograph of the right elbow (*left*) shows marked joint space narrowing, especially at the radiohumeral articulation. Also note the exuberant osteo-

phytes on the ulnar aspect of the articulation. On lateral view (*right*), the nonuniform narrowing of the joint space is more apparent, as are the extensive osteophytes.

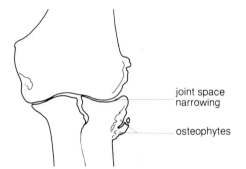

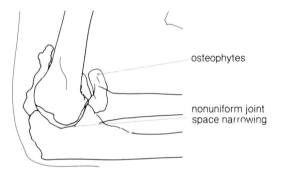

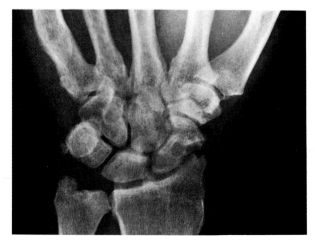

Figure 9.3 Anteroposterior radiograph of the wrist of a jackhammer operator demonstrates marked but nonuniform narrowing of the radionavicular joint space. In addition, the articular surfaces are irregular, and bone cysts are evident within the navicula.

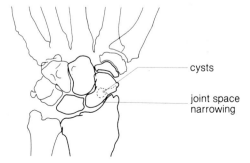

Clinical disease may also occur at atypical sites such as the sternoclavicular (Fig. 9.4), the acromioclavicular (Fig. 9.5), the temporomandibular, and the sacroiliac joints. In the case of the latter two joints, osteoarthritis may present difficult diagnostic problems; therefore, these joints will be discussed in detail later in this chapter.

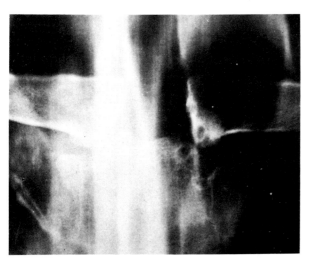

Figure 9.4 Tomogram of the sternoclavicular joint reveals subchondral cysts and sclerosis on both the clavicle and the manubrium of the sternum. These changes are typical radiographic findings in osteoarthritis.

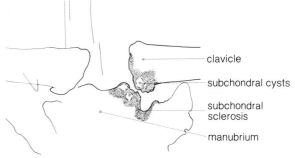

Figure 9.5 Radiograph of the acromioclavicular joint reveals a large osteophyte at the inferior margin, indicating osteoarthritis.

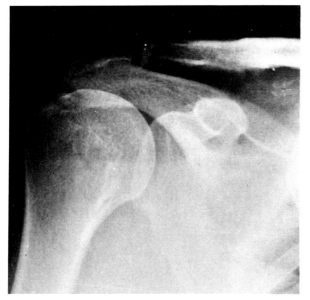

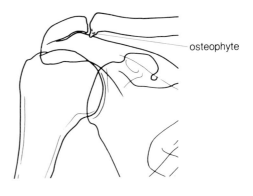

OSTEOARTHRITIS IN ATHLETES

Most physicians have noted an increased incidence of osteoarthritis in athletes and ex-athletes, presumably related to acute and/or chronic injuries. Both the type and incidence of such injuries vary considerably, not only among the different sports but even within a single team. Variables such as degree of physical fitness, muscle development, timing, balance, and skill have been implicated. Adolescents are especially at risk because of their physical immaturity, weakness, hypermobility, and incoordination. It has also been shown that an athlete with a history of previous injury sustains further injury at a significantly higher rate than his fellow athlete without such a history.

In some athletes, osteophytes are seen radiographically without joint space narrowing. This is particularly the case in the ankle joints of football players; radiologic studies have found the majority of changes to consist of rounded or irregular bony outgrowths on the anterior surface of the tibia and talus – and to a lesser extent on the posterior surfaces – without evidence of cartilage degeneration (Fig. 9.6). As previously discussed, bone remodeling occurs constantly throughout life, and bony hypertrophy has been demonstrated experimentally as an effect of running in the rat, and clinically in the dominant arm of professional baseball pitchers and hands of karate experts.

Although osteophytes are often a sign of osteoarthritis, osteophyte formation alone does not indicate cartilage destruction or imply the later development of radiographically demonstrable structural changes. However, certain sports-related joint injuries are clearly related to the later development of osteoarthritis, especially chondromalacia patellae, subluxation and dislocation of the patella, osteochondritis dissecans, synovial effusion with traumatic synovitis, ligamentous injuries, and traumatic meniscal lesions.

Chondromalacia patellae, localized pain over the knee cap, is a diagnosis commonly made in

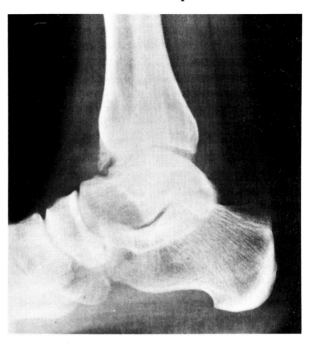

Figure 9.6   Lateral radiograph of the ankle of a football player reveals a large anterior tibial osteophyte which is associated with the player's ankle pain. Although such osteophytes may occur in nonathletes, they are usually asymptomatic.

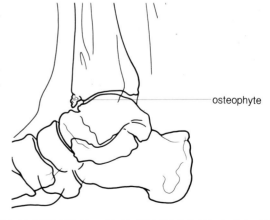

osteophyte

young girls that includes several different types of patellofemoral dysfunction. In most cases it is secondary to patellar subluxation or mild patellar malalignment. Chondromalacia is often found in cyclists and runners due to excessive rotation of the foot, and it may also result from direct trauma. The radiographic changes associated with this condition have already been discussed in Chapter 5 (see Figs. 5.4 and 5.5). Rehabilitation of quadriceps weakness may result in improvement in both clinical and radiographic findings.

Subluxation and dislocation of the patella commonly occur in athletes, with recurrent subluxation ultimately resulting in osteoarthritis of the patellofemoral articulation. Subluxation results from lateral movement of the patella due to angulation between the lines of pull of the quadriceps muscle and the patellar tendon (Q angle, normal less than 15 percent). "Squinting patella syndrome" (Fig. 9.7) frequently occurs in young women, with no relation to physical activity. Treatment consists of exercises designed to strengthen the vastus medialis muscle in order to counteract the lateral movement of the patella. This can be accomplished by repetitive straight leg raising without weights (as many as 300 repetitions). If exercise therapy fails, surgical treatment may become necessary and consists of transposition of the attachment of the patellar tendon to the tibial tubercle so that the lines of pull of the quadriceps and the patellar tendon become the same.

A synovial effusion is often seen after a sports injury and should imply an underlying joint abnormality (Fig. 9.8). An exhaustive search for a remediable mechanical problem is then called for. Diagnosis of traumatic synovitis should be made only by exclusion. Athletes with persistent knee effusion should temporarily refrain from engaging in sports while every effort is made to reduce the effusion and strengthen the quadriceps muscle group. Immediate swelling of the knee joint

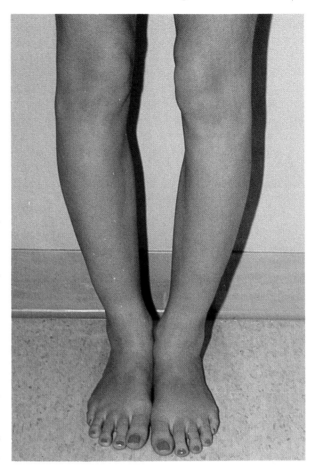

Figure 9.7 Clinical photograph of a patient with "squinting patella syndrome." Femoral anteversion, an increased Q angle, and external tibial torsion cause the patellas to face inward when the feet are together.

after an injury may suggest the presence of blood in the joint. Since blood is much more harmful to the articular cartilage than simple effusion, it is essential to remove as much of the bloody effusion as possible from the joint cavity by arthrocentesis.

Ligamentous injuries are common in most sports and predispose to osteoarthritis. In recent years there has been an emphasis on the early diagnosis and treatment of such injuries, especially of the cruciate ligaments, and surgical repair and reconstruction of these complex ligaments has led to improved joint stability and reduced likelihood of progressive degenerative changes.

Many athletes develop tears of the menisci, and there has been considerable interest in the possible association between meniscectomy and osteoarthritis. Published figures for the incidence of osteoarthritis after meniscectomy range from 23 to 85 percent, but these are based on variable radiologic criteria.

Muscle injuries may also have a direct association with the development of osteoarthritis. Muscles contribute greatly to the stability of some joints, and a reduction in their efficiency allows abnormal movement or instability to occur at the joint with possible damage to the articular surface. Therefore, muscles must be rehabilitated for strength, muscle tone, and endurance.

In review, there does not appear to be an inevitable increased incidence of osteoarthritis with physical activity unless there is a loss of the structural integrity of the joint with a resultant biomechanical defect. Indeed, in a study of 1000 unselected autopsies, Heine (1926) segregated 100 patients who spent many years at hard labor from 100 who did little physical work and found no difference in the incidence of osteoarthritis. Although there is a clear-cut increase in osteophyte formation and bony hypertrophy related to physical activity, the presence of these changes does not necessarily herald the development of structural degenerative changes in the articular cartilage.

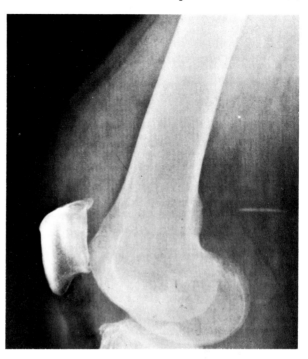

Figure 9.8 Lateral radiograph of the knee shows a large suprapatellar effusion resulting from a sports-related injury.

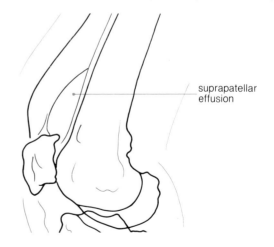

suprapatellar effusion

RUNNING INJURIES

As more and more Americans have taken up running to maintain and/or improve their physical fitness, the incidence of injuries has increased exponentially. Table 9.1 lists the 10 most common running-related injuries which account for about 70 percent of all such injuries. Virtually all running injuries occur in the lower extremity, with the knee being the most common site and accounting for 20 to 40 percent of all injuries. The high incidence of knee injuries probably represents an increase in the ratio of recreational to competitive runners in today's running population.

Patellofemoral pain syndrome is the most common running-related disorder, accounting for almost 30 percent of all such injuries. In general, the causes fall into four categories: training errors, anatomic factors, faulty running shoes, and variable training surfaces.

Training errors include persistent high-intensity training without alternate easy days, sudden increases in training mileage and/or intensity without allowing the supporting structures of the lower extremities sufficient time to adapt to the increased workload, a single severe training or competitive session such as a 10-km race or a marathon, and repetitive hill running.

Anatomic factors include leg-length discrepancy; femoral neck anteversion; quadriceps and hamstring insufficiency; genu valgum, varum, and recurvatum; excessive Q angle (greater than 15°); tibial torsion; patella alta (a high-riding patella); gastrocnemius-soleus muscle insufficiency; and lower-leg–heel and/or heel-forefoot malalignment.

Factors which have been implicated in running shoes are inadequate heel-wedging; soft, loose-fitting heel counters; inflexible soles under the metatarsal heads; narrow toe boxes; excessive lateral heel wear; improper application of sole repair material; and the removal or breakdown of orthoses. Finally, hard surfaces, road camber, and uneven terrain are also occasional etiologic factors.

Table 9.1 Frequency of the 10 Most Common Running-related Injuries

Injury	%
Patellofemoral pain syndrome	26.0
Tibial stress syndrome	13.0
Achilles peritendinitis	6.0
Plantar fasciitis	5.0
Patellar tendinitis	4.5
Iliotibial band friction syndrome	4.0
Metatarsal stress syndrome	3.0
Tibial stress fracture	3.0
Tibialis posterior tendinitis	2.5
Peroneal tendinitis	2.0

ATYPICAL OSTEOARTHRITIS
Temporomandibular Joint Osteoarthritis

Osteoarthritis is the most common type of arthritis which affects the temporomandibular joint. Early symptoms include stiffness in and around the joint upon waking, which disappears with use and returns later in the day. The physical sign of the disease is crepitus, which can be determined by either palpation or auscultation. Other clinical signs include tenderness and pain in the joint. Radiographs reveal narrowing of the joint space, para-articular sclerosis, and osteophyte formation (Fig. 9.9). Temporomandibular osteoarthritis can be distinguished from rheumatoid arthritis by the absence of polyarthritis and the lack of systemic symptoms.

If radiographic evidence of disease is absent, the diagnosis is far more likely to be temporomandibular joint (TMJ) syndrome than osteoarthritis. TMJ syndrome usually occurs in younger individuals who complain of unilateral pain in the ear or in the preauricular area. The pain is usually a constant, dull ache that may radiate to the angle of the jaw, the neck, or the temporal region. The jaw will deviate when opened, indicating muscle spasm with resultant asynchronous movement of the jaw.

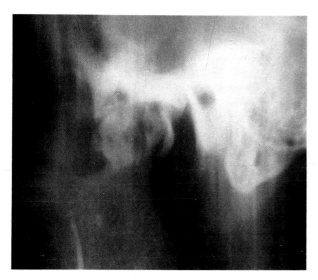

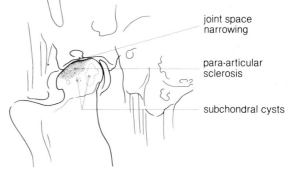

Figure 9.9 Tomogram of the temporomandibular joint reveals joint space narrowing, para-articular sclerosis, and subchondral cyst formation.

joint space narrowing

para-articular sclerosis

subchondral cysts

Sacroiliac Joint Osteoarthritis

The clinical signs of osteoarthritis of the sacroiliac joints are pain in the lower back and tenderness to percussion associated with morning stiffness that is confined to the sacroiliac area. Osteoarthritis is radiologically distinct from sacroiliitis (Fig. 9.10), which occurs in patients with ankylosing spondylitis or the rheumatoid variant diseases (i.e., psoriatic arthritis, Reiter's syndrome, and colitic ar-

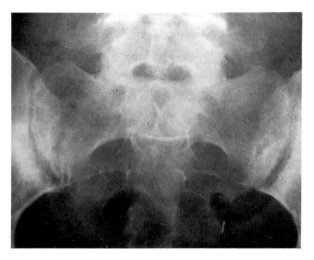
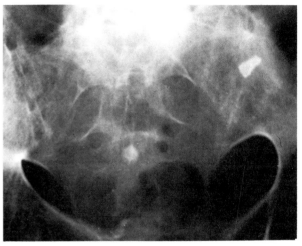

Figure 9.10   Radiograph of the sacroiliac joint in a patient with early ankylosing spondylitis (*left*) demonstrates pseudo-widening of the joint secondary to erosions of the articular cartilage. This widening is referred to as "beading." In a radiograph of more advanced sacroiliitis (specifically, psoriatic arthritis) (*right*), one can observe bridging and ultimately fusion of the sacroiliac joint, a condition associated with extensive osteoporosis.

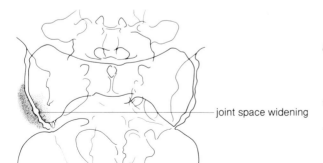
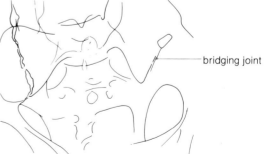

joint space widening

bridging joint

thritis). The radiologic features of osteo-arthritis include irregularity of the joint margin and para-articular sclerosis with sharply defined joint margins (Fig. 9.11). Osteophytes are frequently seen in the lower third of the joint at its most caudad point. In contrast, osteitis condensans ilii is usually an incidental radiographic finding in young women in whom para-articular sclerosis is limited to the iliac side of the sacroiliac joint (Fig. 9.12).

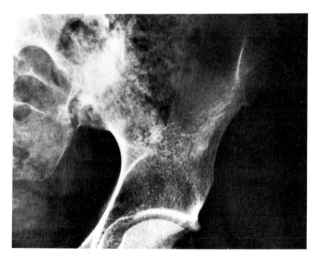

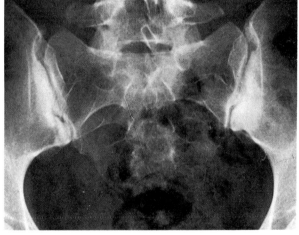

Figure 9.11 Radiograph of the sacroiliac joint in a patient with advanced osteoarthritis shows marked loss of joint space as well as extensive para-articular sclerosis.

Figure 9.12 Radiograph of a patient with osteitis condensans reveals subchondral sclerosis on the iliac aspect of the sacroiliac joint only. The joint space is entirely normal.

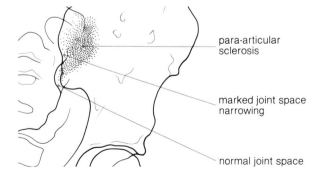

para-articular sclerosis

marked joint space narrowing

normal joint space

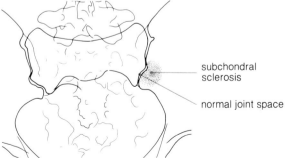

subchondral sclerosis

normal joint space

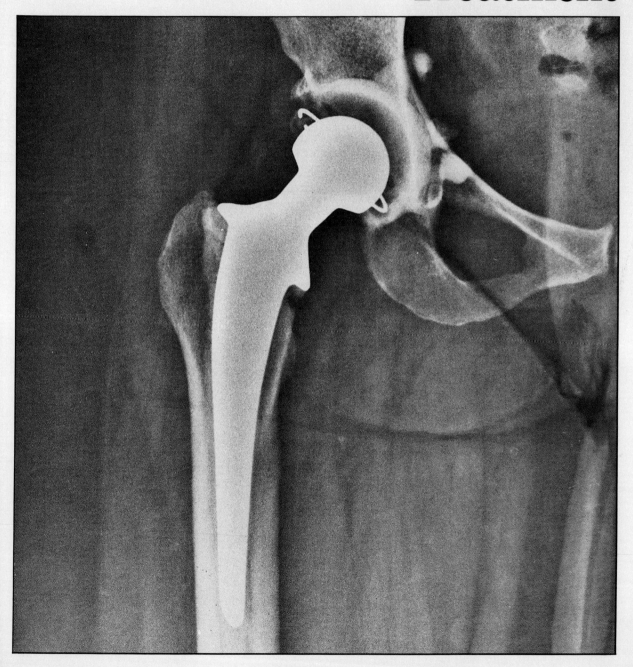

The goal of therapy for patients with osteo-arthritis is alleviation of pain and maintenance of function. There is as yet no definitive treatment that can alter or retard the degenerative process once it has begun. Studies of animals and humans suggest that altering the load or stress on a joint may affect the development and progression of osteoarthritis, particularly in the hip and knee where osteotomy may result in clinical improvement and apparent improvement in the joint space.

Following the diagnosis of osteoarthritis based on clinical and radiographic evidence, the following therapeutic regimen should be applied in a stepwise continuum:

1. The patient should be educated as to the type of arthritis and to its extent. It is important that he or she be reassured that osteoarthritis need not be a crippling disease, and that in the vast majority of cases it does not result in severe disability.

2. Patients should be encouraged to continue their usual daily activities, and to be as active as possible within their own limitations. Progressively increasing range of motion exercises should be prescribed, and in certain situations, monitored physical therapy may be warranted. Appliances such as cervical collars, canes, etc. may be beneficial in some cases.

3. Drug therapy with one of the nonsteroidal anti-inflammatory (NSAI) drugs should be instituted in an attempt to relieve pain. Individual patients may have varying responses to these drugs, and several of these agents may be tried serially to identify the best agent for a given patient.

4. In patients with symptoms disproportionately localized in one joint, and in whom NSAIs have had limited efficacy, the injection of intra-articular corticosteroids may be of some benefit.

5. If the above measures fail to relieve pain and maintain function, surgical debridement or prosthetic replacement of the involved joint may well be indicated.

EDUCATION

Successful therapy requires that the patient understand the goals of management, but the educating process should not be limited to reassurances that the condition is nondebilitating. Many patients must be instructed how to adjust their lifestyles to obtain optimal results.

Although patients can be as active as they wish within their own limitations, periods of rest should be interspersed with periods of activity to give the affected joint time to recover from the stress and strain of activity. For example, it may be helpful to establish a given period of rest in the middle of each day.

Certain physical activities have been found to cause additional trauma and damage when done in excess, and they should therefore be avoided. On the other hand, in patients with osteoarthritis of the hip or knee, swimming provides good exercise without increasing forces on the articular cartilage. Other factors which result in abnormal stress upon the articular cartilage, such as obesity, should be corrected where possible.

PHYSICAL THERAPY

A progressive exercise program should be developed with the individual's needs in mind, and should emphasize improving range of motion as well as strengthening of muscles. Exercises should begin with only one or two repetitions per session and gradually progress. Ultimately, the patient should be able to perform the entire prescribed program without supervision. Used in conjunction with exercise, the application of heat (e.g., hot packs, electric pads, diathermy, or ultrasound) may be helpful in relieving pain and muscle spasm. Note, however, that localized heat may cause or worsen degenerative changes in the articular cartilage, and should be used with caution and directed at the muscle, not at the joint.

In certain cases, the use of appliances may also be appropriate. A cervical collar may be utilized to immobilize the neck in patients with cervical osteoarthritis and radicular pain. Patients should be advised to wear the collar during waking hours, especially when riding in a vehicle or walking for prolonged periods. Weight-bearing joints can be protected by the use of canes, crutches, or a walker. When only one knee or hip is involved, the cane or crutch should be used on the opposite side.

DRUG THERAPY

Nonsteroidal anti-inflammatory (NSAI) drugs are the cornerstone of drug therapy in patients with osteoarthritis (Table 10.1). They may be classified structurally into three groups: (1) the carboxylic acids, which can be further subclassified into the salicylic acids, the propionic

Table 10.1   Dosage and Schedule for Anti-inflammatory Drug Therapy

Drug	Dosage (mg)	Schedule (dosages/day)
Salicylic Acids		
Aspirin	600–900	4
Choline magnesium salicylate	500–1000	2
Salsalate	500–1000	2
Diflunisal	500	2
Propionic Acids		
Ibuprofen	400–800	4
Fenoprofen	200–400	4
Naproxen	250–500	2
Acetic Acids		
Indomethacin	25–50	3
Sulindac	150–200	2
Tolmetin	200–400	4
Fenamic Acids		
Meclofenamic acid	50–100	3
Oxicams		
Piroxicam	20	1

acids, the acetic acids, and the fenamic acids; (2) the pyrazolones; and (3) the oxicams (Fig. 10.1).

Though osteoarthritis is not inherently inflammatory, clinical observations of patients reveal that they show a marked preference for NSAIs over purely analgesic drugs. Some clinicians have proposed that the increased efficacy of anti-inflammatory drugs suggests that perhaps there is an inflammatory component to osteoarthritis. Alternatively, the preference may simply reflect the limited potency of the nonnarcotic analgesics.

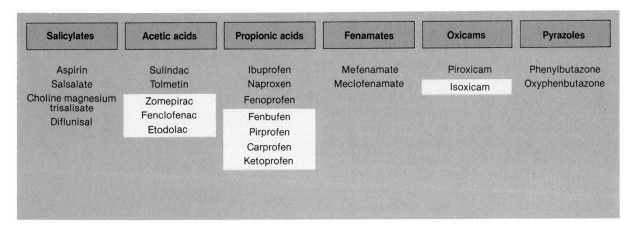

Figure 10.1 Classification of non-steroidal anti-inflammatory drugs. ( ), available in 1984–1985.

In a study of the relative therapeutic efficacy of various analgesics in patients with cancer (before the advent of the newer agents), aspirin — the prototype anti-inflammatory drug — proved superior to placebo and to most of the other agents tested, including acetaminophen, propoxyphene, and codeine (Fig. 10.2).

Since osteoarthritis may be characterized by quiescent periods, the use of anti-inflammatory drugs may be required only intermittently, as needed for relief of pain. In patients with persistent pain, drugs may have to be administered regularly in an ongoing course of therapy. Aspirin is the time-honored anti-inflammatory drug, and although there has been a recent proliferation of newer agents, a trial of aspirin therapy may be warranted for some patients with osteoarthritis. (It should be noted that recent data suggest that aspirin may actually impede cartilage repair and consequently hasten the degenerative process. This may explain the recent willingness of clinicians to prescribe one of the newer nonsteroidals rather than aspirin as a first-line drug.)

Aspirin (600 to 1200 mg) may be taken in anticipation of pain by patients with osteoarthritis of the hip, knee, or first MTP joint of the foot if prolonged walking or standing is likely to exacerbate pain. For individuals with chronic pain, aspirin may be required in doses of 600 to 900 mg four times a day.

The most common adverse effect of aspirin — and all anti-inflammatory drugs for that matter — is gastric intolerance, which manifests as epigastric discomfort, nausea, or anorexia. The ingestion of aspirin causes gastric erosions and occult blood loss from the gastrointestinal tract in the majority of patients, but this blood loss rarely results in significant anemia. Tinnitus and decreased auditory acuity are early and reliable signs of salicylate toxicity in adults. In young adults, tinnitus usually occurs at serum salicylate levels ranging from 20 to 30 mg/dl. In children, the serum salicylate level required to cause tinnitus may be much higher, or tinnitus may not occur at all. Although tinnitus is commonly found in patients taking salicylate, ototoxicity is entirely reversible.

Serious adverse reactions to aspirin are uncommon, with anaphylaxis occurring in only 0.2 percent of patients. However, a clinical syndrome of nasal polyps and asthma has been found to occur in some patients with aspirin hypersensitivity. Decreased glomerular filtration rates have been reported in patients with underlying renal disease. Elevations of hepatic enzymes may be transient, and they may return to normal even when aspirin administration is continued.

Several preparations of aspirin have been marketed with an enteric coating to decrease gastrointestinal adverse reactions. Newer preparations of salicylate such as choline magnesium salicylate, salsalate, and diflunisal may be as effective as aspirin, with less accompanying gastrointestinal intolerance and bleeding. In addition, these preparations can be administered in simple, twice-daily doses.

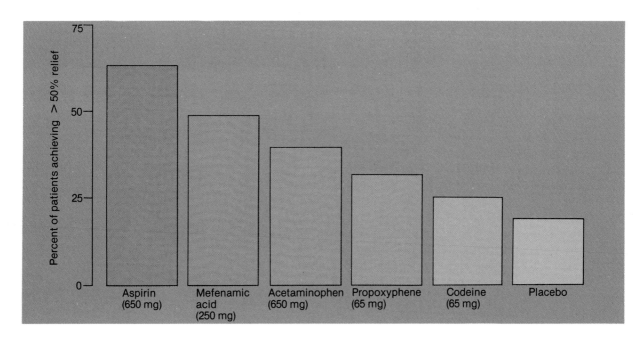

Figure 10.2   Relative therapeutic effect of oral analgesics for patients with cancer. (From Moertel et al., 1972)

Newer anti-inflammatory drugs are now available for patients with osteoarthritis. The propionic acid derivatives, having less gastrointestinal toxicity, were developed as an alternative to aspirin. Compared to aspirin, these drugs result in a marked decrease in the percentage of patients who develop gastric ulcerations (Fig. 10.3). Fenoprofen and ibuprofen have plasma half-lives of about 2 hours and must be administered four times daily. Fenoprofen (1.8 to 2.4 g/day) is effective in the treatment of osteoarthritis, with improvement in symptoms occurring in 60 to 80 percent of patients. Ibuprofen (400 mg) is roughly equivalent in potency to 600 mg of aspirin. Naproxen has a longer half-life than the aforementioned drugs; given in doses of 250–500 mg twice daily, naproxen has been found to be more effective than placebo and comparable to indomethacin in patients with osteoarthritis of large joints. Fenbufen is yet another propionic acid derivative that may be available shortly in the U.S.

Indomethacin is the prototype of the heterocyclic acetic acids, and along with aspirin is the standard against which newer anti-inflammatory drugs are compared. It may be more effective than aspirin in some patients, and is a reasonable alternative for those patients who cannot tolerate aspirin. Indomethacin and tolmetin must be given three or four times daily; however, a newer preparation of indomethacin has a sustained release and may therefore be administered only twice daily. Since the active metabolite of sulindac has a half-life of 16 to 18 hours, this drug may also be administered twice daily. Sulindac has been found to be more effective than placebo and as effective as aspirin in the treatment of osteoarthritis; it is more effective than ibuprofen (1200 mg daily) in osteoarthritis of the hip.

Studies have found that the heterocyclic acetic acids may be associated with more severe gastrointestinal adverse effects than are found with aspirin. Of patients receiving indomethacin, 2 to 5 percent develop bleeding ulcers, and 10 to 25 percent experience central nervous system effects, the latter incidence apparently increasing with age. Patients may experience morning frontal headaches, vertigo, feelings of dissociation or unreality, depression, hallucinations, or psychosis. These central nervous system symptoms may be avoided by starting therapy at low dosages and increasing the dosages by small increments, or by the administration of drugs only at bedtime. Central nervous system toxicity appears to occur less often after therapy with sulindac and tolmetin.

Although marketed as an analgesic, zomepirac (400 mg/day) is an acetic acid derivative which is useful alone or in combination with NSAIs in the treatment of osteoarthritis. While it is generally well-tolerated, it does present similar side effects to other NSAIs, including severe allergic reactions, and has been removed from the market in the U.S. It may be reapproved for limited usage in patients with intractable pain unresponsive to other analgesics.

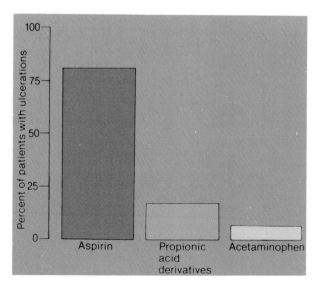

Figure 10.3 Frequency of erosive or ulcerative lesions of the gastric mucosa in patients taking propionic acid derivatives as compared to aspirin and acetaminophen.

The phenylacetic acids — diclofenac and alclofenac — are not yet available in the United States, but the European experience suggests that these drugs may be as effective as the heterocyclics but with fewer adverse effects.

The fenamic acids are halogenated anthranilic acid derivatives that provide a new therapeutic option for those patients who have not responded to other drugs. Meclofenamate (50 to 100 mg) is administered in three divided doses, but up to a third of patients on a full regimen of the drug have been found to develop diarrhea.

The oxicams are characterized by high potency and a long half-life, allowing once-daily administration. Piroxicam has been shown to be significantly superior to aspirin in reducing pain in osteoarthritic joints. In 20-mg doses, piroxicam results in about the same gastrointestinal disturbances and other adverse effects as the propionic acid derivatives, though significantly less frequently than with aspirin. Similar results have also been found with isoxicam.

The pyrazolones — phenylbutazone and its major metabolite, oxyphenbutazone — have been available for more than 20 years. However, because of the incidence of serious side effects such as aplastic anemia, pancytopenia, and granulocytopenia, and the current availability of newer, less toxic NSAIs, the pyrazolones are no longer warranted for the treatment of osteoarthritis.

Purely analgesic drugs such as acetaminophen and propoxyphene may be used in combination with nonsteroidal anti-inflammatory drugs, but their contribution to the therapeutic efficacy of NSAIs is questionable. Narcotic analgesics have no place in the treatment of osteoarthritis because of the potential of habituation and dependency.

OTHER FORMS OF TREATMENT

In rare situations where one joint is considerably more involved than the others or where there is an obvious inflammatory reaction taking place, the use of intra-articular corticosteroids may prove beneficial. Caution is advised because repeated injections may actually hasten the degenerative process, especially in weight-bearing joints, and Charcot's joints may occur.

Various corrective surgical procedures have played a major role in the ongoing management of the patient with osteoarthritis. At various points in the disease process, the following procedures may be performed: surgical debridement of the joint with or without removal of loose bodies; arthrodesis (fusion of the joint), osteotomy to alter joint mechanics, and total joint replacement. Clinical data suggest that osteotomy may lead to improvement in the joint and regeneration of cartilage, especially in the hip and knee.

In cases where degeneration is severe, total joint replacement procedures may be warranted. Prostheses of the hip have been found to be especially effective in older patients (see Chapter 4). In younger patients, however, the accumulated wear products of the prostheses may cause a significant synovitis. Although prosthetic knees, ankles, and shoulders are available, they are currently less highly developed and, consequently, less successful than hip prostheses.

Bibliography

Acheson RM, Collart AB: New Haven survey of joint diseases. XVII. Relationship between some systemic characteristics and osteoarthrosis in a general population. Ann Rheum Dis 34: 379, 1975.

Adams ID: Sports injury and osteoarthrosis. Practitioner 224: 61, 1980.

Adams ID: Osteoarthrosis and sport. J Soc Health 72: 185, 1979.

Adams ME, Billingham MEJ, Muir H: The glycosaminoglycans in menisci in experimental and natural osteoarthritis. Arth Rheum 26: 69, 1983.

Ahlbäck S: Osteoarthrosis of the knee; a radiographic investigation. Acta Radiol Suppl 277: 1, 1968.

Ali SY, Bayliss T: Enzymic changes in human osteoarthritic cartilage. In Ali SY, Elves MW, Leaback DH (eds.) Normal and Osteoarthrotic Articular Cartilage. London, Institute of Orthopaedics, 1974, p. 189.

Bennett GA, Waine H, Bauer KW: Changes in the Knee Joint at Various Ages with Particular Reference to the Nature and Development of Degenerative Joint Disease. New York, The Commonwealth Fund, 1942.

Bird HA, Tribe CR, Bacon PA: Joint hypermobility leading to osteoarthrosis and chondrocalcinosis. Ann Rheum Dis 37: 203, 1978.

Bland JH, Stulberg SD: Osteoarthritis: Pathology and clinical patterns. In Kelley WN et al. (eds.) Textbook of Rheumatology, vol. 2. Philadelphia, Saunders, 1981, pp. 1471–1490.

Bluestone R, Bywaters EGL, Hartog M et al.: Acromegalic arthropathy. Ann Rheum Dis 30: 243, 1971.

Bollet AJ: An essay on the biology of osteoarthritis. Arth Rheum 12: 152, 1969.

Bollet AJ: Connective tissue polysaccharide metabolism and the pathogenesis of osteoarthritis. Adv Intern Med 13: 33, 1967.

Bollet AJ, Nance JL: Biochemical findings in normal and osteoarthritic cartilage. II. Chondroitin sulfate concentration and chain length, water and ash contents. J Clin Invest 45: 1170, 1966.

Bollet AJ, Handy JR, Sturgill BC: Chondroitin sulfate concentration and protein polysaccharide composition of articular cartilage in osteoarthritis. J Clin Invest 42: 853, 1963.

Brandt KD: Pathogenesis of osteoarthritis. In Kelley WN et al. (eds.) Textbook of Rheumatology, vol. 2. Philadelphia, Saunders, 1981, pp. 1457–1470.

Brandt KD: Proteoglycans: Structure and metabolism. Arth Rheum (Suppl) 20: S109, 1977.

Brandt KD, Palmoski M: Organization of ground substance proteoglycans in normal and osteoarthritic knee cartilage. Arth Rheum 19: 209, 1976.

Brooks PM, Potter SR, Buchanan WW: Editorial: NSAID and osteoarthritis - help or hindrance? J Rheum 9: 3, 1982.

Broom J: Obesity: Its relationship to osteoarthritis. Clin Orthopaed Rel Res 93: 271, 1973.

Bullough PG: The geometry of diarthrodial joints. Its physiologic maintenance, and the possible significance of age related changes in geometry to load distribution and the development of osteoarthritis. Clin Orthopaed Rel Res 156: 61, May 1981.

Bullough PG: Some considerations of chronic hip disease and its treatment. J Ir Col Phys Surg 8: 43, 1978.

Bullough PG, Walker PS: The distribution of load through the knee joint and its possible significance to the observed patterns of articular cartilage breakdown. Bull Hosp Joint Dis 37: 110, 1977.

Bullough PG, Goodfellow JW, Greenwald AS et al.: Incongruent surfaces in the human hip joint. Nature 217: 1290, 1968.

Burke MJ, Fear EC, Wright V: Bone and joint changes in pneumatic drillers. Ann Rheum Dis 36: 276, 1977.

Cailliet R: Neck and Arm Pain. Philadelphia, Davis, 1977.

Chrisman OD, Snook GA, Wilson TC: The protective effect of aspirin against degeneration of human articular cartilage. Clin Orthopaed Rel Res 84: 193, 1972.

Clement DB, Tauton JE, Smart GW, McNicol KL: A survey of overuse running injuries. Phys Sportsmed 9: 47, 1981.

Cooper NS, Soren A, McEwen C: Diagnostic specificity of the synovial lesions. Hum Pathol 12: 314, 1981.

Crock HV: Post-traumatic erosions of articular cartilage. J Bone Joint Surg 46B: 530, 1964.

Danielsson L, Hernborg J: Clinical and roentgenologic study of knee joints with osteophytes. Clin Orthopaed Rel Res 69: 302, 1970.

Danielsson L, Hernborg J: Morbidity and mortality of osteoarthritis of the knee (gonarthrosis) in Malmö, Sweden. Clin Orthopaed Rel Res 69: 224, 1970.

Detenbeck LG, Tressler HA, O'Duffy JD et al.: Peripheral manifestations of acromegaly. Clin Orthopaed Rel Res 91: 119, 1973.

Dieppe PA et al.: The inflammatory component of osteoarthritis. In Nuki G (ed.) The Etiopathogenesis of Osteoarthrosis. London, Pittman Medical, 1980, pp. 117–122.

Dolman CL, Bell HM: The pathology of Legg-Calvé-Perthes disease. A case report. J Bone Joint Surg 55A: 184, 1973.

Ehrlich GE: Osteoarthritis beginning with inflammation. JAMA 232: 157, 1975.

Ehrlich MG, Mankin HJ, Jones H, Wright R, Crispen C, Vigliani G: Collagenase and collagenase inhibitors in osteoarthritic and normal human cartilage. J Clin Invest 59: 226, 1977.

Engel A: Osteoarthritis and body measurements. United States 1960–1962, U.S.

Public Health Service Bull., Washington, D.C., Ser. 11, No. 29, 1968.

Engel A, Burch TA: Osteoarthritis is adults by selected demographic characteristics: United States 1960–1962. U.S. Public Health Service Bull., Washington, D.C., Ser. 20, No. 11, 1966.

Fell HB, Jubb RW: The effect of synovial tissue on the breakdown of articular cartilage in organ culture. Arth Rheum 20: 1359, 1977.

Feller ER, Schumacher HR: Osteoarticular changes in Wilson's disease. Arth Rheum 15: 259, 1972.

Freeman MAR: The fatigue of cartilage in the pathogenesis of osteoarthrosis. Acta Orthopaed Scand 46: 323, 1975.

Freeman MAR: Discussion on pathogenesis of osteoarthrosis. In Ali SY, Elves MW, Leaback DH (eds.) Normal and Osteoarthrotic Articular Cartilage. London, Institute of Orthopaedics, 1974, pp. 301–319.

Glynn LE: Primary lesion in osteoarthrosis. Lancet 1: 574, 1977.

Gofton JP, Trueman, GE: Studies of osteoarthritis of the hip. Part II. Osteoarthritis of the hip and leg length disparity. Can Med Assoc J 104: 791, 1971.

Goldenberg DL, Eagen MS, Cohen AS: Inflammatory synovitis in degenerative joint disease. J Rheumatol 9: 204, 1982.

Goldin RH, McAdam L, Louie JS et al.: Clinical and radiological survey of the incidence of osteoarthrosis among obese patients. Ann Rheum Dis 35: 349, 1976.

Goodfellow JW, Bullough PG: The pattern of aging of the articular cartilage of the elbow. J Bone Joint Surg 49B: 175, 1967.

Harris ED Jr., Parker HG, Radin EL, Krane S: Effects of proteolytic enzymes on structural and mechanical properties of cartilage. Arth Rheum 15: 497, 1972.

Heine J: Über die arthritis deformans. Virchows Arch [Path Anat] 260: 521, 1926.

Hjertquist SO, Lemperg R: Identification and concentration of the glycosaminoglycans of human articular cartilage in relation to age and osteoarthritis. Calcif Tissue Res 10: 223, 1971.

Hjertquist SO, Wasteson A: The molecular weight of chondroitin sulphate from articular cartilage. Effect of age and osteoarthritis. Calcif Tissue Res 10: 31, 1972.

Howell DS: The pathogenesis of osteoarthritis. Sem Arth Rheum 5: 365, 1976.

Howell DS, Moskowitz RW: Symposium on osteoarthritis. Arth Rheum (Suppl) 20: S96, 1977.

Howell DS, Pita JC, Sorgente N et al.: Possible role of lysozyme in degradation of osteoarthritic cartilage. Trans Assoc Am Phys 87: 169, 1974.

Howell DS, Sapolsky AI, Pita JC, Woessner JF: The pathogenesis of osteoarthritis. Sem Arth Rheum 5: 365, 1976.

Huskisson EC et al.: Another look at osteoarthritis. Ann Rheum Dis 38: 423, 1979.

Inerot S, Heinegard D, Audell L, Olsson S: Articular cartilage proteoglycans in aging and osteoarthritis. Biochem J 169: 143, 1978.

Insall J (ed): Surgery of the Knee. New York, Churchill Livingstone, 1984.

James SL, Bates BT, Osternig LR: Injuries to runners. Amer J Sports Med 6: 40, March–April 1978.

Johnson LC: Joint remodelling as a basis for osteoarthritis. J Am Vet Med Assoc 141: 1237, 1962.

Jorring K: Osteoarthritis of the hip: Epidemiology and clinical role. Acta Orthopaed Scand 51: 523, 1980.

Kellgren JH, Lawrence JS: Osteoarthrosis and disk degeneration in an urban population. Ann Rheum Dis 17: 388, 1958.

Kellgren JH Lawrence JS: Radiological assessment of osteoarthrosis. Ann Rheum Dis 16: 494, 1957.

Kellgren JH, Moore R: Generalized osteoarthritis and Heberden's nodes. Brit Med J 1: 181, 1952.

Kellgren JH, Ball J, Tutton GK: The articular and other limb changes in acromegaly: A clinical and pathological study of 25 cases. Q J Med 21: 405, 1952.

Krissoff WB Ferris WD: Runners' injuries. Phys Sportsmed 7: 55, December 1979.

Kuettner KE, Harper E, Eisenstein R: Protease inhibitors in cartilage. Arth Rheum (Suppl) 20: S124, 1977.

Lane LB, Villacin A, Bullough PG: The vascularity and remodelling of subchondral bone and calcified cartilage in adult human femoral and humoral heads. J Bone Joint Surg 59B: 272, 1977.

Lawrence JS: Generalized osteoarthrosis in a population sample. Amer J Epidemiol 90(5): 381, 1969.

Lawrence JS, Brenner JM, Bier F: Osteoarthrosis: Prevalence in the population and relationship between symptoms and x-ray changes. Ann Rheum Dis 25: 1, 1966.

Leach RE, Baumgard S, Broom J: Obesity: Its relationship to osteoarthritis of the knee. Clin Orthopaed Rel Res 93: 271, June 1973.

Lee P, Rooney PJ, Sturrock RD, Kennedy AC, Dick WC: The etiology and pathogenesis of osteoarthrosis: A review. Sem Arth Rheum 3: 189, 1974.

Lippiello LL, Hall D, Mankin HJ: Collagen synthesis in normal and osteoarthritic human cartilage. J Clin Invest 59: 593, 1977.

McCarty DJ: Calcium pyrophosphate dihydrate crystal deposition disease: Nomenclature and diagnostic criteria. Ann Intern Med 87: 241, 1977.

McDevitt CA: Biochemistry of articular cartilage. Nature of proteoglycans and collagen of articular cartilage and their role in aging and osteoarthrosis. Ann Rheum Dis 32: 364, 1973.

McMaster MJ: The pathogenesis of hallus rigidus. J Bone Joint Surg 60B: 82, 1978.

Macys JR, Bullough PG, Wilson PD: Coxarthrosis: A study of the natural history based on a correlation of clinical, radiographic and pathologic findings. Sem Arth Rheum 10 (1): 66, August 1980.

Mankin HJ: The reaction of articular cartilage

to injury and osteoarthritis. N Engl J Med 291: 1335, 1974.

Mankin HJ, Lippiello L: The glycosaminoglycan of normal and arthritic cartilage. J Clin Invest 50: 1712, 1971.

Mankin HJ, Thrasher AZ, Hall D: Biochemical and metabolic characteristics of articular cartilage from osteonecrotic human femoral head. J Bone Joint Surg 59A: 724, 1977.

Marmor L, Peter JB: Osteoarthritis of the hand. Clin Orthopaed Rel Res 64: 164, 1969.

Maurer K: Basic data on arthritis. Knee, hip and sacroiliac joints in adults ages 25–74 years, United States, 1971–1975. DHEW publications 79–1661, Ser. 11, No. 213, August 1979.

Muir H: Molecular approach to the understanding of osteoarthrosis. Ann Rheum Dis 36: 199, 1977.

Nichols EH, Richardson FL: Arthritis deformans. Med Res 21: 149, 1909.

Nimni ME: Collagen: Its structure and function in normal and pathological connective tissues. Sem Arth Rheum 4: 95, 1974.

Oldberg S: On the etiology of Heberden's nodes. Upsala J Med Sci 83: 43, 1978.

Palmoski MJ, Brandt KD: Aspirin aggravates the degeneration of canine joint cartilage caused by immobilization. Arth Rheum 25: 1333, 1982.

Palmoski MJ, Brandt KD: Effect of salicylate on proteoglycan metabolism in normal canine articular cartilage in vitro. Arth Rheum 22: 746, 1979.

Palmoski MJ, Coyer RA, Brandt KD: Marked suppression by salicylate of the augmented proteoglycan synthesis in osteoarthritic cartilage. Sem Arth Rheum 23: 83, 1980.

Pelletier J, Martel-Pelletier J, Howell DS, Ghandur-Mnaymneh L, Enis JE, Woessner JF Jr.: Collagenase and collagenolytic activity in human osteoarthritic cartilage. Arth Rheum 26: 63, 1983.

Peter JB, Pearson CM, Marmor L: Erosive osteoarthritis of the hands. Arth Rheum 9: 365, 1966.

Peyron JG: Epidemiologic and etiologic approach of osteoarthritis. Sem Arth Rheum 8(4): 288, May 1979.

Polley HF, Hunder GG: Rheumatologic Interviewing and Physical Examination of the Joints, 2nd ed. Philadelphia, Saunders, 1978.

Radin EL: Aetiology of osteoarthritis. Clin Rheum Dis 2: 509, 1976.

Radin EL: Mechanical aspects of osteoarthritis. Bull Rheum Dis 26: 862, 1976.

Radin EL: The physiology and degeneration of joints. Sem Arth Rheum 2: 245, 1972–1973.

Repo RU, Finlay JB: Survival of articular cartilage after controlled impact. J Bone Joint Surg 59A: 1068, 1977.

Roberts J, Burch TA: Prevalence of osteoarthritis in adults by age, sex, race, and geographic area, United States, 1960–1962. Public Health Service Bull, Washington, D.C., Ser. 11, No. 15, June 1966.

Sapolsky AI, Altman RD, Howell DS: Cathepsin D activity in normal and osteoarthritic human cartilage. Fed Proc 32: 1489, 1973.

Sapolsky AI, Howell DS, Woessner JF Jr.: Neutral proteases and cathepsin D in human articular cartilage. J Clin Invest 53: 1044, 1974.

Saville PD, Dickson J: Age and weight in osteoarthritis of the hip. Arth Rheum 11: 635, 1968.

Silberberg M, Silberberg R: Role of sex hormones in the pathogenesis of osteoarthrosis of mice. Lab Invest 12: 285, 1963.

Smukler NM, Edeiken J, Giuliano VJ: Ankylosis in osteoarthritis of the finger joints. Radiology 100: 525, 1971.

Sokoloff L: Pathology and pathogenesis of osteoarthritis. In McCarty DJ (ed.) Arthritis and Allied Conditions, 9th ed. Philadelphia, Lea & Febiger, 1979, pp. 1135–1153.

Sokoloff L: The Biology of Degenerative Joint Disease. Chicago, University of Chicago Press, 1969.

Solomon L: Patterns of osteoarthritis of the hip. J Bone Joint Surg 58B: 176, 1976.

Stephens RW, Ghosh P, Taylor TKF: The pathogenesis of osteoarthritis. Med Hypotheses 5: 809, 1979.

Twersky J: Joint changes in idiopathic hemochromatosis. Am J Roentgenol Rad Ther Nucl Med 124(1): 139, May 1975.

Venn MR: Variation of chemical composition with age in human femoral head cartilage. Ann Rheum Dis 37: 168, 1978.

Waine H, Nevinny D, Rosenthal J et al.: Association of osteoarthritis and diabetes mellitus. Tufts Folia Med 7: 13, 1961.

Walton M: Obesity as an aetiological factor in the development of osteoarthritis. Gerontology 25: 36, 1979.

Weightman BO, Freeman MAR, Swanson SAV: Fatigue of articular cartilage. Nature 244: 303, 1973.

Yazici H, Saville PD, Salvati EA et al.: Primary osteoarthrosis of the knee or hip. Prevalence of Heberden's nodes. JAMA 231: 1256, 1975.

Index

Reiter's disease, **3.1t**
Reiter's syndrome
 and joint fluid findings, **2.2t**
 and sacroiliitis, 9.10
Rheumatic fever, **2.2t**
Rheumatoid arthritis
 and cervical disk disease, 7.12, **7.12**
 hand, **3.1t**
 and joint fluid findings, **2.2t**
 and knee pain, **5.1t**
 and neck pain, **7.1t**
 and osteoarthritis classification, **2.3t**
 and protrusio acetabuli, 4.10
 and synovial membrane injury, 1.19, **1.32**
Rib clavicle compression, **7.1t**
Rotation, cervical spine, 7.6–7.7, **7.6**
Running injuries, **9.1t**, 9.8
Running shoes, 9.8

S
Sacralization, 8.17, **8.21**
Sacroiliac joint, 9.4, 9.10–9.11, **9.10–9.12**
Sacroiliitis, 9.10–9.11, **9.10**
Salicylic acids, **10.1t**
Salsalate, **10.1t**, 10.7
Sarcoid arthritis, **3.1t**
Scalene muscle, and neck pain, **7.1t**
Schmorl's nodes, 8.14, **8.16**
Sciatic pain, 8.8
Scleroderma, 2.2t
Sclerosis
 discogenic, 8.13, **8.14**
 first metatarsophalangeal joint, **6.4**
 hand, **3.1t**
 knee, 5.17, **5.19, 5.20**
 para-articular sclerosis. **See** Para-articular sclerosis
 subchondral, **2.6, 2.9**
  and chondromalacia patellae, **5.5**
  and sacroiliac joint, **9.12**
  shoulder, **9.1**
Sclerotic bone, and osteochondritis dissecans, **5.3**
Scoliosis, lateral, 8.9
Secondary osteoarthritis, **2.2t**, 4.10–4.14
Septic arthritis, **2.3t**
Septic spondylitis, **7.1t**
Sex, 1.27–1.28, **1.41**
Sex hormone abnormalities, **2.3t**
Shoulder-hand syndrome, 7.9
Shoulder osteoarthritis, **9.1**, 9.2
 incidence of, **2.12**
Sickle cell anemia, 2.16, 4.14
Slipped capital femoral epiphysis, 2.12, **2.14**, 4.10, 4.12, **4.12**
Spasm, lumbar, 8.9

Spinal cord compression, 7.9
Spinal stenosis, **8.2t**
Spondylitis
 ankylosing, **7.1t**
  and hand, **3.1t**
  and joint fluid findings, **2.2t**
  and low back pain, **8.2t**
  and neck pain, **7.1t**
  and sacroiliitis, 9.10
 septic, **7.1t**
Spondyloarthritides
 and hand, **3.1t**
 and osteoarthritis classification, **2.3t**
Spondylolisthesis, degenerative, **8.2t**, 8.16, **8.19, 8.20**
Spondylosis, and low back pain, **8.2t**
Sports-related injuries. **See** Athletes; Running injuries
Squinting patella syndrome, 9.6, **9.7**
Standing posture evaluation, 8.9
Steinmann's tenderness displacement sign, 5.14, **5.15**
Stenosis
 lateral, 8.7
 spinal, **8.2t**
Sternoclavicular joint, **9.4**
Steroid therapy
 and osteoarthritis classification, **2.3t**
 and osteonecrosis, **2.3t**
Straight leg raising test, 8.10, **8.12**
 and nerve root impingement, **8.1t**
Structural defects, 1.30
Subchondral cysts, 3.10, **3.12**
 first metatarsophalangeal joint, 6.4, 6.6
 hip joint, 4.9, **4.10, 4.11**
Subchondral necrosis, 2.13, **2.18–2.20**
Subluxation, knee, 5.18, **5.20**
Sulindac, **10.1t**, 10.8–10.9
Suprapatellar effusion, knee, **9.8**
"Swayback," **8.3**, 8.4
Synovial effusions, knee, 5.15
Synovial fluid, **2.1t, 2.2t**
Synovial membrane injury, 1.19–1.20
 hyperplasticity, **1.31**
 hypertrophy, **1.31**
 rheumatoid arthritis and, **1.32**
 synovial membrane extension, **1.33**
Synovitis, traumatic, 9.6

T
Talonavicular joint osteoarthritis, 6.9, **6.15**
Tarsal joint osteoarthritis, 6.8–6.9, **6.14**
Temporomandibular joint, 9.4, 9.9, **9.9**
Temporomandibular joint syndrome, 9.9
Tendon reflexes, 8.11
 and nerve root impingement, **8.1t**
Tibial torsion, 9.8